# Gimel Review
# NMC CBT Practice
# Questions and Answers.

Elaine Matthew RN, BSN.

# GIMEL'S INTRODUCTION

**GIMEL** Comprehensive Self Study Program!
In this book you shall find pattern of questions as in the actual
NMC CBT test.

It contains over 300 practice questions and answers which
comprises of different sections of NMC Study guide topics. These
are: *Assessment and Discharge planning; Communication;
Infection Prevention and Control; Laboratory Diagnostics
and Test; Leadership in Nursing; Medicines Management;
Moving and Positioning; Nutrition, Fluid balance and Blood
Transfusion; Observation; Patient Comfort and End of Life
Care; Patient Safety; Pre-operative Care; Psychosocial Care;
Respiratory Care; Vulnerable Adult and Children; Wound
Management.*
It will help you gain strong confidence and fully be prepared for
this test.
Also get a copy of **"Gimel Review for the NMC CBT test", or
the updated edition of the same title. "Gimel Review for the
NMC CBT test, Updated Edition", by the same author.**
Go through the review contents and then practice more questions
in this book that covers over NMC CBT 300 practice questions
and answers.

Give yourself maximum of three weeks of daily concentrated two
hours of studies. Go through the review book or the eBook and
then test your knowledge with these questions and answers.

Whether this is your first attempt or you have attempted this test
several times. I want to encourage you to stay focused on your
goals and you will surely achieve this success.

# Table of Contents

# NMC CBT PRACTICE TEST QUESTIONS.

# Assessment and Discharge Planning

1. The nurse is providing discharge teaching for a client with newly diagnosed Crohn's disease about dietary measures to implement during exacerbation episodes. Which of these statements made by the clients indicates lack of understanding of the instructions?
   A. "I will need to avoid caffeinated drinks".
   B. "I should increase the fiber in my diet".
   C. "I can have exacerbations and remissions with Crohn's disease".
   D. "I'm going to learn some stress reduction".

2. Which is not included in the intermediate care?
   A. Maximize dependent living.
   B. Prevent unnecessary acute hospital admission.
   C. Prevention of premature admission to long term residential care.
   D. Support timely discharge from hospital.

3. A client with CVA is found to have difficulty in swallowing. Whom do you think should be informed for further assessment?
   A. Neurological Physiotherapist.
   B. Occupational Physiotherapist.
   C. Speech Therapist.
   D. Physical Therapist.

4. **For every patient admitted in the ward, discharge planning should be done at which time of the process?**
   A. Within 24 hours of admission.
   B. When patient tells he wants to leave.
   C. When the family request for a discharge.
   D. Immediately after the doctor's order for discharge.

5. **While gaining consent the nurse should assess for _____ ability of the patient.**
   A. Capacity.
   B. Understanding.
   C. Emotions.
   D. Sensitivity.

6. **Which is the most suitable site for assessing oedema?**
   A. Foot/Ankle.
   B. Clavicle.
   C. Sternum.
   D. Scapular.

7. **A patient is assessed for lacking capacity to give consent if they are unable to _____. (*Choose several Options*).**
   A. Understand information about the decision and remember that information.
   B. Use that information to make a decision.
   C. Communicate their decision by talking, using sign language or by any other means.
   D. The patient is unconscious.

8. **Common causes for hyperglycaemia includes all of the following except: (*Choose several options*).**
   A. Not eating enough protein.
   B. Deficiency of Insulin.
   C. Infection.
   D. Stress.

9. **What is AVPU?**
   A. A replacement for GCS.
   B. An assessment for confusion.
   C. Assessment for the level of consciousness.
   D. Monitor the level of unconsciousness.

10. **On assessment of the abdomen of a patient with peritonitis you would expect to find:**
   A. Rebound tenderness and guarding.
   B. Hyperactive, high-pitched bowel sounds and a firm abdomen.
   C. A soft abdomen with bowel sounds every 2 to 3 seconds.
   D. Ascites and increased vascular pattern on the skin.

11. **Most patients with gastric ulcers typically exhibit which of the following symptoms:**
   A. Epigastric pain worsens before meals, pain awakening patient from sleep and melena.
   B. Decreased bowel sounds, rigid abdomen, rebound tenderness, and fever.
   C. Boring epigastric pain radiating to back and left shoulder, bluish-grey discoloration of periumbilical area and ascites.
   D. Epigastric pains worsens after eating and weight loss.

12. **Which of the following would indicate an infection?**
   A. Hot, sweaty, a temperature of $36.5^0C$, and bradycardia.
   B. Temperature of $38.5^0C$, shivering tachycardia and hypertensive.
   C. Raised WBC, elevated blood glucose and temperature of $36.0^0C$.
   D. Hypertensive, cold and clammy, and bradycardia.

13. **What should be included when carrying out initial assessment of a patient's respiratory status?**
    A. Review the patient's notes and charts, to obtain the patient's history.
    B. Review the results of routine investigations.
    C. Observe the patient's breathing for ease and comfort, rate and pattern.
    D. Perform a systematic examination and ask the relatives for the patient's history.

14. **What would make you suspect that a patient in your care had a urinary tract infection?**
    A. The doctor has requested a midstream urine specimen.
    B. The patient has a urinary catheter in situ and the patient's wife states that he seems more forgetful than usual.
    C. The patient has spiked in temperature, has a raised white blood cell (WBC), and in a confused state and the urine in their catheter bag is cloudy.
    D. The patient has complained of frequency of faecal elimination and hasn't been drinking enough.

15. **A patient was diagnosed to have Crohn's disease. Among the following which are the signs and symptoms?** *Choose several options.*
    A. Blood and mucous in the faeces.
    B. Fatigue.
    C. Loss of appetite.
    D. Diarrhea.

16. **Which of the following is a risk factor when assessing the causes of falling in older adults?**
    A. Slight tremors.
    B. Some medications.
    C. Atrophy of muscles and strength.
    D. All of the above.

17. **Which statement is not correct about the nursing process?**
    A. An organized, systematic and deliberate approach to nursing with the aim of improving standards in nursing care.
    B. It uses a systematic, holistic, problem solving approach in partnership with the patient and their family.
    C. It is a form of documentation.
    D. It requires collection of objective data.

18. **When doing your shift assessment, one of your patient has a waterlow score of 20. Which of the following mattress is appropriate for this score?**
    A. Fluidized airbed.
    B. Waterbed.
    C. Low air loss.
    D. Alternating pressure.

19. **What is the main objectives in providing stoma education when preparing a patient with a stoma for discharge home?**
    A. That the patient can independently manage their stoma, and can get supplies.
    B. That the patient has had their appliance changed regularly, and knows their community stoma nurse.
    C. That the patient knows the community stoma nurse, and has a prescription.
    D. That the patients has a referral to the district nurses for stoma care.

20. **When do you see potential problems in a client or patient?**
    A. Assessment.
    B. Diagnosis.
    C. Implementation.
    D. Evaluation.

**21.** **What may not be the cause of diarrhea?**
A. Colitis.
B. Intestinal obstruction.
C. Food allergy.
D. Food poisoning.

# Communication

22. According to Argyle (1988), when two people communicates, the percentage in words and not the body language is?
    A. 23%
    B. 90%
    C. 50%
    D. 7%

23. In non-verbal communication, what does SOLER stand for?
    A.    Squarely, open posture, leaning slightly forward, eye contact, relaxed.
    B.    Squarely, open ended questions, leaning slightly forward, eye contact, relaxed.
    C. Squarely, open posture, leaning forward, eye contact, rested.
    D. Squarely, open ended questions, leaning slightly backwards, rested.

24.   What are the key competences and features for effective collaboration?
    A. Effective communication skill, mutual respect, constructive feedback and conflict management.
    B. High level of trust and honesty, giving and receiving feedback, and decision making.
    C. Mutual respect and open communication, critical feedback, cooperation, and willingness to shear ideas and decisions.
    D. Effective communication and decreased competition for scares resource.

25. **What are the characteristics of effective collaboration?**
    A. Common purpose and goals
    B. Clinical competence of each provider
    C. Humor, trust, and valuing diverse, complementary knowledge
    D. All of the above

26. **What are the essential skills for current nurse managers?**
    A. A vision and goals
    B. Communication and tem work.
    C. self and group awareness
    D. Strategic planning and design.

27. **Which of these is the most appropriate therapeutic communication?**
    A. I'm sorry, your mother died.
    B. I'm sorry, your mother has gone to Heaven.
    C. I'm sorry, your mother is no longer with us.
    D. I'm sorry, your mother passed away.

28. **There is a Chinese client in your care and the relatives of the client insisted on bringing their own food for the client, what is the appropriate things for the nurse to do?**
    A. Accept their wishes under Western Foods and Cultural differences considerations.
    B. Refuse the client's wish as the food might carry infection.
    C. Ask the next of kin to bring in the food and hand it to the dietary unit for approval.
    D. Tell them it is not accepted, firmly.

29. A patient suffered from stroke and is unable to read and write. This is called?
   A. Dysphasia.
   B. Dysphagia.
   C. Partial aphasia.
   D. Aphasia.

30. The nurse can divulge patients information, only when
   A. It becomes a threat to the public and when it is ordered by the court
   B. The media insists for disclosure.
   C. Relating in a professional manner.
   D. Communicating effectively.

31. Which of the following are barriers to effective communication?
   A. Unfamiliar ascent.
   B. Overly technical language and terminology.
   C. Hearing problems.
   D. All of the above.

32. What factors are essential in demonstrating supportive communication to patients?
   A. Listening, clarifying the concerns and feelings of the patient using open questions.
   B. Listening, clarifying the physical needs of the patient using closed questions.
   C. Listening, clarifying the physical needs of the patient using open questions.
   D. Listening, reflecting back the patient's concerns and providing a solution.

33.     **Which of the following is not an example of non-verbal communication.**
   A. Dress.
   B. Facial expression.
   C. Posture.
   D. Tone.

34.     **What are the principles of communicating with a patient with delirium?**
   A. Use shot statements and closed questions in a well-lit, quiet and familiar environment.
   B. Use short statements and open questions in a well-lit, quiet and familiar environment.
   C. Write down all questions for the patient to refer back to.
   D. Communicate only through the family using short statement and closed questions.

35.     **When communicating with someone who is not a native English speaker, which of the following is not advisable?**
   A. Using a translator.
   B. Use short precise sentences.
   C. Relying on their family of friends to explain what you mean.
   D. Write things down.

36.     **Which of these is an example of an open question?**
   A. Are you feeling better today?
   B. When you said you are hurt, what do you mean?
   C. Can you tell me what is concerning you?
   D. Is that what you are looking for?

37. A nurse is to establish a rapport with the patient and family, elements of the history include all the following except:
    A. The client's health status.
    B. The course of the present illness.
    C. Social history.
    D. Cultural beliefs and practices.

38. When a nurse communicates with children. What should be the best consideration?
    A. Developmental level.
    B. Physical development.
    C. Parental involvement.
    D. Nonverbal cues.

39. During which part of the client interview would it be best for the nurse to ask, "What's the weather forecast for today?"
    A. Introduction.
    B. Body.
    C. Closing.
    D. Orientation.

40. Which behaviour will encourage a patient to talk about their concerns?
    A. Giving reassurance & telling them not to worry.
    B. Asking the patient about their family & friends.
    C. Tell the patient you are interested in what is concerning them & that you are available to listen and to keep it confidential.
    D. Tell the patient you are interested in what is concerning them if they tell you, they will feel better.

41. **How do you give respect and dignity to your client as a nurse?**
    A. Compassion, support & reassurance to the client.
    B. Giving advice on health care issues.
    C. Relating in a professional manner.
    D. Communicating effectively.

42. **Which of the steps is not involved in Tuckman's formation theory?**
    A. Accepting.
    B. Forming.
    C. Norming.
    D. Storming.

# Infection prevention and control

43. Which of the following indicates an infection?
    - A. Hot, diaphoresis, 36.5°c and bradycardia.
    - B. Shivering, 38.4°c, tachycardia and hypertensive.
    - C. Elevated blood glucose, 36.2°c, Elevated WBC.
    - D. Hypotensive, bradycardia, cold and clammy body.

44. A relative of a patient talks to the nurse over the phone and asks permission to come and visit the patient in the hospital. She admitted that she had few episodes of vomiting and diarrhea. What is the best response by the nurse?
    - A. Don't allow her to come and meet the patient.
    - B. Ask her to come and visit after 48hrs of recovery from the symptoms.
    - C. Advise her to sanitize the hands with hand sanitizer.
    - D. Advise her to treat herself.

45. How do you take an infected sheet for washing according to the UK standard?
    - A. Take infected linen in yellow bag for disposal.
    - B. Take in the red plastic bag that disintegrates in high temperature.
    - C. Use red linen bag that allows washing in high temperature.
    - D. Take the linen to the laundry.

46. A patient with Clostridium difficile has bloody mucoid stool due to which of the following conditions?
    - A. Ulcerative colitis.
    - B. Crohn's disease.
    - C. Inflammatory bowel disease.
    - D. Colitis.

**47.** *Which of these notifiable diseases needs to be reported on a national level? Choose several options.*
   A. Chicken pox.
   B. Tuberculosis.
   C. Whooping cough.
   D. Influenza.

**48.** **Examples of offensive/hygiene waste which may be sent for energy recovery at energy waste facilities include:**
   A. Stoma or catheter bags.
   B. Unused non-cytotoxic/cytostatic medicines in original packaging.
   C. Used sharps from treatment using cytotoxic or cytostatic medicines.
   D. Empty medicine bottles.

**49.** **What infection control steps should not be taken in a patient with diarrhea caused by Clostridium Difficile?**
   A. All staff will be required to wash their hands before and after contact with the patient, their bed linen and soiled items.
   B. Isolation of the patient.
   C. All staff must wear aprons and gloves while attending the patient.
   D. None of the above.

**50.** **The use of an alcohol-based hand rub for decontamination and clinical care is recommended when?**
   A. Hands are visibly soiled.
   B. Caring for patients with vomiting or diarrhea illness, regardless of whether or not gloves have been worn.
   C. Before and immediately after contact with patients, body fluids, mucous membranes and non-intact skin.
   D. Hands are cleaned with Napkin.

51. **You were told a patient in your care had 'Source Isolation'. What would you do and why?**
    A. Isolating a patient so that they are not infected.
    B. Nursing an individual who is regarded as being particularly vulnerable to infection in such a way as to minimize the transmission of potential pathogens to that person.
    C. Nurse the patient in isolation, ensure that you wear appropriate personal protective equipment (PPE) and adhere to strict hand hygiene, for the purpose of preventing the spread of organisms from that patient to others.
    D. Nursing a patient who is carrying an infectious agent that may be a risk to others in such a way as to minimize the risk of the infection spreading elsewhere in their body.

52. **What steps would you take if you had sustained a needle stick injury?**
    A. Ask for advice from the emergency department, report to occupational health and fill in an accident form.
    B. Gently make the wound bleed, place under running water and wash thoroughly with soap and water. Cover any wound with a waterproof dressing to prevent entry of any other foreign material. Complete an incident form and inform your manager. Co-operate with any action to screen yourself or the patient for infection with blood borne virus but do not obtain blood or consent for testing from the patient yourself; this should be done by someone not involved in the incident.
    C. Take blood from patient and self for Hepatitis B screening and take samples and form to Bacteriology. Call your union representative for support. Make an appointment with your GP for a sick leave certificate and take time off until the wound site has healed so you don't contaminate any other patients.

D. Wash the wound with soap and water. Cover any wound with a waterproof dressing to prevent entry of any other foreign material

53. **MRSA means?**
    A. Methilinase Resistant Streptococcus Aureus.
    B. Methicillin Resistant Streptococcus Aureus.
    C. Methilinase Resistant Staphylococcus Aureus.
    D. Methicillin Resistant Staphylococcus Aureus.

54. **Define Standard precaution:**
    A. The precautions that are taken with all blood and 'high-risk' body fluids.
    B. The actions that should be taken in every care situation to protect patients and others from infection, regardless of what is known of the patient's status in regard to infection.
    C. It is meant to reduce the risk of transmission of blood Bourne and other pathogens from both recognized and unrecognized sources.
    D. The practice of avoiding contact with bodily fluids, by means of wearing of nonporous articles such as gloves, goggles, and faces shields.

55. **Which client has the highest risk of a bacteremia?**
    A. Client with a peripherally inserted central catheter (PICC) line.
    B. Client with a Central venous catheter (CVC).
    C. Client with an implanted infusion port.
    D. Client with a peripherally inserted intravenous line.

56. **Prions causes infection known as** _____
    A. Pneumonia.
    B. Measles.
    C. Creutzfeldt- jakob.
    D. None of the above.

57.     When disposing of waste, what colour of bag should be
        used to dispose of offensive/hygiene waste?
        A. Orange.
        B. Yellow.
        C. Yellow and black stripe.
        D. Black.

58.     Hand hygiene is a key preventative measure for which
        of the following modes of transmission?
        A. Airborne.
        B. Direct & indirect contact.
        C. Droplet.
        D. All of the above.

59.     The following procedures required all nurses providing
        care to be competent with except?
        A. Hand hygiene.
        B. Use of protective equipment.
        C. Disposal of waste.
        D. Aseptic technique.

# Laboratory Diagnostics and Tests

60. The expected signs and symptoms of a patient with Crohn's disease are the following except:
   A. Fever, diarrhea, anorexia, anemia, weight loss, colicky pains after eating, dehydration, electrolytes imbalance and malnutrition.
   B. Fever, anorexia, anemia, constipation, electrolytes imbalance and malnutrition.
   C. Fever, diarrhea, constipation, electrolytes imbalance, Colicky pains after eating, dehydration, Weight loss and malnutrition.
   D. None of the above.

61. In Interpreting ECG results, there is clear evidence of atrial disruption. This is interpreted as?
   A. Cardiac arrest.
   B. Ventricular tachycardia.
   C. Atrial fibrillation.
   D. Complete blockage of the heart.

62. A patient in your care is about to go for a liver biopsy. What are the most likely potential complications of this this procedure?
   A. Inadvertent puncture of pleural, a blood vessel or bile duct.
   B. Inadvertent puncture of the heart, oesophagus or spleen.
   C. Cardiac arrest requiring resuscitation.
   D. Inadvertent of the kidney and cardiac arrest.

63. Prothrombin time is essential during anticoagulation therapy. In oral anticoagulation therapy which of the test is essential?
   A. Activated Thromboplastin Time.
   B. International Normalized Ratio.
   C. Hematocrit.
   D. Hemoglobin.

64. If a patient feels cramping sensation in their abdomen after colonoscopy, it is advisable that they should do or have which of the following?
   A. Eat fluid based food or low residue diet and or drink more of fluid to avoid dehydration as soon as sedation has worn off.
   B. Be nursed flat and kept in bed for 12 hours.
   C. Drink 500ml of fluid immediately to flush out any gas retained in the abdomen.
   D. Have half hourly blood pressure perform for 12 hours.

65. Which of the following is not an indication for Lumbar tap?
   A. Introduction of contrast medium.
   B. Spinal anesthesia for surgery.
   C. For patients with increased ICP
   D. For diagnostic purposes.

66. How do you ensure the correct blood culture ratio, when obtaining a blood culture specimen from an adult patient?
   A. Collect blood until specimen bottle stops filling.
   B. Collect at least 5mL of blood.
   C. Collect at least 10mL of blood.
   D. Collect as much blood as possible.

67. If a patient should have a pacemaker in-situ, which of the following diagnostics will not be allowed to be done?
   A. Barium swallow.
   B. CT scan.
   C. MRI.
   D. X-ray.

**68.** **If blood sample is required to be taken for various other test from a patient, which should come first to reduce the risk of contamination?**
A. Take the other blood test first.
B. Inoculate the anaerobic culture first.
C. The order does not matter as long as the bottles are clean.
D. Inoculate the aerobic culture first.

**69.** **What are the contraindications for the use of blood glucometer for blood glucose monitoring?**
A. The patient has needle phobia and prefer to have a urinalysis.
B. If the patient is in a critical care setting, the staff will send venous sample to the laboratory for verification of blood glucose level.
C. If the device has not been calibrated.
D. If peripheral circulation is impaired, collection of capillary blood is not advised, as the result might not be a true reflection of the physiological blood glucose level.

**70.** **If a patient is experiencing dysphagia, which of the following investigations his likely to have?**
A. Gastroscopy
B. Arthroscopy
C. Colonoscopy
D. Cystoscopy.

# Leadership in Nursing

**71. Clinical audit is best describe as:**

   A.   A tool to evaluate the effectiveness of interventions and to know what needs to be improved.

   B.   A standard in which performance is best upon.

   C.   A tool to set guidelines or protocol in clinical practice.

   D.   A tool used to identify the weakest link within the system.

**72.  The contingency theory of management moves the manager away from which of the following approaches?**

   A.   No perfect solution.

   B.   One size fits all.

   C.   Interaction of the system with the environment.

   D.   A method or combination of methods that will be most effective in a given situation.

**73.  If a nurse manager achieves a higher management position in the organization, what types of skills is needed?**

   A. Personal and communication skills.

   B. Communications and technical skills.

   C. Conceptual and interpersonal skills.

   D. Visionary and interpersonal skill.

**74. Transformational leadership is characterized by all of the following elements except?**

   A. Charisma.

   B. Inspirational leadership.

   C. Intellectual stimulation.

   D. Incentives to promote loyalty and performance.

75. **Which nursing delivery model is based on a production of efficiency model which stresses a tax oriented approach?**
    A. Case management
    B. Primary nursing
    C. Differentiated practice
    D. Functional method

76. **If a patient has been assessed and observed that he lacks capacity to make their own decision, what government legislation or 'act' should he be referred to?**
    A. Health and social care act (2012)
    B. Mental capacity act (2005)
    C. Carers (equal opportunities) act (2004)
    D. All of the above.

77. **The nurse manager of a health care facility wishes to prepare and develop nurse managers to several new units that the organization will open next year. What should be the primary goal of this role?**
    A. Focus on rewarding current staff for doing a good job.
    B. Train these managers for them to focus on maintaining standards of care
    C. Prepare these managers to oversee the entire health care organization.
    D. Prepare these managers to interact with hospital administration.

78. **A patient says, "I hate this cancer". According to Kubbler Ross stages of dying, the nurse understand that statement to refer as :**
    A. Anger.
    B. Denial.
    C. Depression.
    D. Bargaining.

79. **A Community Hospital in a local place should provide, what services?**
    A. Rehabilitation, Physiotherapy, Psychiatry, Acute care.
    B. Rehabilitation, Respite care, Acute and primary care, Physiotherapy, Psychiatry, Occupational therapy, Palliative care, Step down care for discharged patients.
    C. Rehabilitation, Acute and Primary care, Occupational therapy, Step down care for discharged patients.
    D. Rehabilitation, Respite care, Palliative care, Step down care for discharged patients.

80. **A Community health nurse is taken history with the second year nursing student in a patient home. The nurse notice that a student nurse is not interested in the group discussion but was chatting on her phone. What is the ideal response from the Community health nurse?**
    A. Ask the student to leave the group.
    B. Caution her at that moment by letting her know that such behaviour is not acceptable.
    C. Inform to the principal.
    D. Talk to her privately and let her be aware that such behavior is not expected of nurses.

81. **You are the nurse at the Community care centre. An elderly patient complained to you that his neighbor is stealing money from him. He spends it on his shopping and sometimes the neighbor does not shop but rather keeps the money with him. What will you do?**
    A. Confront the neighbor when he visit you next time.
    B. Remain quiet and ignore the complaint.
    C. Request that the elderly talk to the Hospital Chaplin for further assistance.
    D. Raise the complaint in the incident report form and investigate the matter as well as inform the concerned authorities.

82. **A mentally disordered client wants to leave the hospital. The medical team is not happy with his clinical condition according to the Mental Health Act. What is your next action?**
    A. Let the client leave the hospital as long as he does not possess any threat to the public or visibly ill.
    B. Inform the security to hold the patient and do not let him go away.
    C. Inform the police.
    D. Counsel the patient to stay back in the hospital for him to get much better.

83. **What is the purpose of Clinical Audit?**
    A. It helps to understand the functioning and effectiveness of nursing activities.
    B. Helps to understand the outcomes and process of medical and surgical procedures.
    C. Helps to identify areas of improvement in the system pertaining to Nursing and medical practitioner.
    D. Helps to understand medical outcomes and process only.

84. **What is Independent Advocacy?**
    A. Providing general advice.
    B. Making decisions for someone.
    C. Agreeing with everything a person says and doing anything a person asks you to do.
    D. None of the above.

85. **In Independent Mental Capacity Advocates (IMCA), when will IMCA make a decision for the client?**
    A. When there is a close family member.
    B. When there is a close friend.
    C. When there is intermittent mental illness in patient.
    D. When there is no friend and family present to make a wish or take a decision for the client.

86. **As a registered nurse what step would you take to guide a new registered nurse who is confused and does not want to make assumptions on patients care, in order to give effective care in accordance to the Code 2005?**
    A. Promote professionalism and trust.
    B. Prioritize people.
    C. Practice effectively.
    D. Promote safety.

87. **You can delegate medication administration to a student if?**
    A. The student was assessed as competent.
    B. Only under close and direct supervision.
    C. The patient has only oral medication.
    D. The student has had administered such medications several times.

88. **What is the purpose of the NMC code?**
    A. It outlines specific tasks or clinical procedures.
    B. It ascertains in detail nurses or midwives clinical expertise.
    C. It is a tool for educating and registering prospective nurses and midwives.
    D. It gives details information on educational programme.

89. **NMC requires in UK how many units of continuing education units a nurse should have in 3 years?**
    A. 35 units.
    B. 45 units.
    C. 55 units.
    D. 65 units.

90. **You are to take charge of the next shift of nurses. Few minutes before your shift, the head nurse in charge of the current shift informed you that two of your nurses will be absent. Since there is a shortage of staff in your shift, what will you do?**
    A.  Encourage all the staff who are present to do their best to attend to the needs of the patients.
    B.  Ask from your manager if there are qualified staff from the previous shift that can make up the number for your shift while you try to replace with new nurses to cover up.
    C.  Refuse to take charge of the next shift.
    D.  Document and do the best you can within your scope.

91. **Whom do you report first if there is a shortage of supplies in your shift?**
    A.  Nursing assistant.
    B.  Purchasing personnel.
    C.  Immediate nurse manager.
    D.  Supplier.

92. **Under the Carers (Equal opportunities) Act (2004) what are Carers entitled to?**
    A.  Their own assessment.
    B.  Financial support.
    C.  Respite care.
    D.  All of the above.

93. **What is accountability?**
    A.  It means that individuals are responsible for their actions and maybe asked to justify them.
    B.  It is intelligent kindness and is central to how people perceive their care.
    C.  It means all those in caring roles must have the ability to understand an individual's health and social needs.
    D.  It enables us to do the right thing for the people we care for.

94. **Which law provides communication aid to patient with disability?**
    A. Communication Act.
    B. Equality Act.
    C. Mental Capacity Act.
    D. Children and Family Act.

95. **What is Advocacy according to NHS Trust?**
    A. It is taking action to help people say what they want, secure their rights, represent their interests and obtain the services they need.
    B. This is the divulging or provision of access to data.
    C. It is the response to the suffering of others that motivates a desire to help.
    D. It is set of rules or a promise that limit access or places restrictions on certain types of information.

96. **What is the primary focus of a nurse manager in a Unit?**
    A. Developing the most effective teams.
    B. Taking risks.
    C. Routine work.
    D. Understanding the history of the organization.

97. **A very young nurse has been promoted to be the nurse manager of an in-patient surgical unit. The nurse is concerned that older nurses may not respect the manager's authority because of the age difference. How can she effectively exercise authority?**
    A. Use critical thinking to solve problems on the unit.
    B. Give assignments clearly, taking staff expertise into consideration.
    C. Understand complex health care environments.
    D. Maintain an autocratic approach top influence results.

98. **A nurse has just been promoted to be a unit manager. What advice, offered by a senior unit manager, will help this nurse become inspirational and motivational in this new role?**
    A. "If you make a mistake with your staff, admit it, apologize, and correct the error if possible."
    B. "Don't be too soft on the staff. If they make mistake, be certain to reprimand them immediately."
    C. "Give your best nurses attention and rewards for their help."
    D. "Never get into a disagreement with a staff member."

99. **Role conflict can occur in any situation in which nurses' work as a team. The major reason for role conflict to emerge in any collaboration is because people have different:**
    A. Levels of education and preparation.
    B. Expectations about a particular role; interpersonal conflicts will emerge.
    C. Levels of experience and exposure of working in interdisciplinary teams.
    D. Values, beliefs, and work experiences that influence their ability to collaborate.

100. **Today many individuals are seeking answers for acute and chronic health problems through non-traditional approaches to health care. What are two popular choices being selected by health consumer?**
    A. Mindful awareness techniques and medication practice.
    B. Stress management and biofeedback programs.
    C. Support groups and alternative medicine.
    D. Tele health and the internet.

101. **A person supervising a nursing student in the clinical area is called?**
   A. Mentor
   B. Interceptor
   C. Supervisor
   D. Preceptor

102. **As a nurse, you are supervising a 3rd year student and you asked her to dispense medication to your patient. What will your assessment be?**
   A. If she is able to administer the medicine.
   B. That she has the understanding of the procedure.
   C. That she is competent and have required skills.
   D. Supervise directly.

103. **The nurse is leading an in-service Continuing education about management issues. The nurse would intervene if another nurse made which of the following statement?**
   A. "It is my responsibility to ensure that the consent form has been signed and attached to the patient's chart prior to surgery".
   B. "It is my responsibility to witness the signature of the client before surgery is performed.
   C. "It is my responsibility to answer questions that the patient may have prior to surgery".
   D. "It is my responsibility to provide a detailed description of the surgery and ask the patient to sign the consent form".

104. **The Nursing and Midwifery regulatory body in the UK with the aim to protect the health & well-being of the public is:**
   A. GMC.
   B. NMC.
   C. BMC.
   D. WHC.

105. Among the following values incorporated in NMC's 6C's, which is not included?
   A. Commitment.
   B. Confidentiality.
   C. Courage.
   D. Care.

106. The Principles of Management (14 in number) was first defined by:
   A. James Watt.
   B. Adams Smith.
   C. Henry Fayol.
   D. Elton Mayo.

## Medicines Management

107. A patient was prescribed metformin 1000mg twice a day for his diabetes. While talking with the patient he stated "I did not eat breakfast so I took half of the tablet at lunch and a whole tablet at super because I don't want my blood sugar to drop." As his primary care nurse you should:

A. Tell him he has made good decision and to continue.
B. Tell him to make a whole tablet with lunch and with super.
C. Tell him to skip the morning dose and just take the dose at super.
D. Tell him to take one tablet in the morning and one tablet in the evening as ordered.

108. What does the term "breakthrough pain" mean, and what type of prescription would you expect for it? *Choose several options.*

A. A patient who has adequately controlled pain relief with short-lived exacerbation of pain, with a prescription that has no regular time of admission of analgesia.
B. Pain on movement which is short-lived, with a prescription, when necessary.
C. Pain that is intense, unexpected in a location that differs from the previously assessed, needing a review before a prescription is written.
D. A patient who has adequately controlled pain relieve with short-lived exacerbation of pain, with a prescription that has 4-hourly frequency of analgesia if necessary.

**109.** The nurse is about to give digoxin tablet to a patient. And she noticed that the patient's heart rate was 58 beats per minute. What is your next action?
A. Give the medication because it is prescribed.
B. Give the medication as patient says this is his normal range of heart rate.
C. Hold the medication, document and report.
D. Hold the medication and beep the doctor.

**110.** A patient is on sub cute Fentanyl skin patch, common side effect of the Fentanyl overdose is:
A. Fast and deep breathing, dizziness, sleepiness.
B. Slow and shallow breathing, dizziness, sleepiness.
C. Noisy and shallow breathing, dizziness, sleepiness.
D. Wheezes and shallow breathing, dizziness, sleepiness.

**111.** A medication of 150g was prescribed and it is available as 5g per tablet. How many tablets are needed to be administered?
A. 30 tablets.
B. 15 tablets.
C. 3 tablets.
D. 5 tablets.

**112.** While changing the tubing on a patient with central line on the right subclavian what should the nurse do to prevent complication?
A. Ask patient to breath normally.
B. Ask patient to hold the breath and bear down.
C. Inhale slowly.
D. Exhale slowly.

113. A new staff was careless about documenting patient's information and was reported by her colleague. What will be your action in solving this issue as the nurse manager?
  A. Make her contact with the person that did the induction programme.
  B. Advice the colleague to help her.
  C. In private call the staff and enquire about the problems in the new job area and give clarifications as it is very important because it may affect the patient's care.
  D. Report her carelessness to the Board.

114. A drug 75ml is to be infused over half an hour. Calculate the milliliters in an hour.
  A. 150m/hr.
  B. 100m/hr.
  C. 75m/hr.
  D. 50m/hr.

115. A drug 8.25mg is ordered, it is available as 2.75mg. Calculate the dosage.
  A. 2 tablets
  B. 3 tablets
  C. 1 tablet
  D. 4 tablets

116. Paracetamol 1gm is ordered but it is available as 500mg. How many tablets is needed to be administered?
  A. 2 tablets.
  B. 5 tablets.
  C. 1 tablet.
  D. 3 tablets.

117.   **When a doctor does prescribed a broad spectrum antibiotics?**
A. On admission.
B. When the blood culture shows positive growth from organisms.
C. After obtaining blood samples for culture.
D. During medication administration.

118.   **What type of drugs causes most of the falls in older patients?**
A. Hypnotics.
B. Loop diuretics.
C. Beta blockers.
D. Non-steroidal anti-inflammatory drugs.

119.   **The proper eye administration installation position is**
A. Supine.
B. Sit up and head tilt backwards.
C. Sit up and lean forward.
D. Standing.

120.   **The important advice that should be given to a patient on medication (allopurinol) should be to?**
A. Drink plenty of fluid.
B. Take analgesics.
C. Take whenever patient demand for it.
D. Give with herbal preparation.

121. **You are caring for a Hindu client and it's time for drug administration, the client refuses to take the capsule saying that animal products might have been used in producing the drugs, what is the appropriate action for the nurse to perform?**
   A. She will not administer but document the omissions in the patients chart.
   B. The nurse will ignore the clients request and administer forcefully.
   C. The nurse will open the capsule and administer the powdered drug.
   D. The nurse will have to collaborate with the pharmacist to determine if the capsule is suitable for vegetarians.

122. **A nurse is performing covert administration of drugs to the client, which of the following is an appropriate explanation of this?**
   A. Convert administration of drugs to clients is ethically and professionally wrong.
   B. Assess the deprivation of liberty, safeguards and mental capacity of the client and then administer in accordance with the multi-disciplinary team care plan.
   C. Convert administration of drugs can only be allowed if the client's next of kin advises so.
   D. Give without the patient's consent.

123. **Adequate record keeping for a medical device should provide evidence for?**
   A. A unique identifier for the device, where appropriate.
   B. A full history, including date of purchase and where appropriate when it was put into use, deployed or installed.
   C. Any specific legal requirements and whether these have been met.
   D. All of the above.

124. The doctor prescribes a dose of 9mg of an anticoagulant for a patient being treated for thrombosis. The drug is being supplied in 3mg a tablet. How many tablets should you administer?
   A. 3 tablets.
   B. 1.5 tablets.
   C. 6 tablets.
   D. 9 tablets.

125. The doctor prescribes 25mg of a drug to be given by injection. It is a drug dispensed in a solution strength of 50mg/ml. How many mL should you administer?
   A. 2m.
   B. 1.5ml.
   C. 0.5ml
   D. 2.5ml.

126. A doctor prescribes an injection of 200 micrograms of drug. The stock bottle contains 1mg/ml. How many ml will you administer?
   A. 20ml.
   B. 2ml.
   C. 0.2ml.
   D. 1ml.

127. Under the Yellow Card Scheme which of the following is a concern and must be reported to.
   A. Faulty brakes on a wheelchair.
   B. Suspected side effects to blood factor, except immunoglobulin products.
   C. Counterfeit or fake medicines or medical devices.
   D. Incident report.

128. **Which colour contain medical waste for incineration?**
    A. Blue bag
    B. Orange waste bag, before being placed in the appropriate linen bag, no more than a quarter full.
    C. White linen bag, after sorting, no more than a quarter full.
    D. Yellow Polythene bag.

129. **What could be the reason for instructing your patient to retain its original container and to discard nitroglycerine medication after 8 weeks?**
    A. Removing from its darkened container exposes the medicine to light and its potency will decrease after 8 weeks.
    B. It will have a greater concentration after 8 weeks.
    C. It will protect the effect.
    D. It will decrease its concentration.

130. **Which is the most dangerous site for intramuscular injection?**
    A. Ventrogluteal.
    B. Deltoid.
    C. Rectus femoris.
    D. Dorsogluteal.

131. **On which step of the World Health Organisation Analgesic ladder would you place tramadol and codeine?**
    A. Step 1: Non-Opioid Drugs.
    B. Step 2: Opioids for mild to moderate pain.
    C. Step 3: Opioids for moderate to severe pain.
    D. Herbal Medicine.

132. **Which medicine does digoxin interact with?**
    A. NSAID.
    B. Rasagiline.
    C. Amoxicillin.
    D. Anticoagulants.

133. **Before administering Digoxin, you must check specifically for what?**
    A. Breathing.
    B. Temperature.
    C. Heart Rate.
    D. Level of consciousness.

134. **What are the most common types of medication error?**
    A. Unsafe handling and poor aseptic technique.
    B. Doctors not prescribing correctly and poor communication with the multidisciplinary team.
    C. Nurses being interrupted when completing their drug rounds, different drugs being packaged similarly and stored in the same place with calculation errors.
    D. Administration of the wrong drug, in the wrong amount, to the wrong patient and or through the wrong route.

135. **Select the option that do not apply. How should nurses transfer controlled drugs?**
    A. A person collecting controlled drugs should be aware of safe storage, the importance of handling it over to authorized person(s) in other to obtain their signature and be security alert.
    B. Controlled drugs should be transferred in a secure locked or sealed, tamper- proofed evident container.
    C. Have valid ID badge.
    D. None of the above.

136. **When do we need document?**
    A. As soon as possible after an event has happened to provide current up to date information about the care and condition of the patient or client.
    B. Every hour.
    C. When there are significant changes to the patient's condition.
    D. At the end of the shift.

137. **What are the indications for pleural tubing?**
*Choose several options.*
   A. Malignant pleural effusion.
   B. Pneumothorax.
   C. Post- operative conditions such as thoracotomy, cardiac surgery.
   D. Abnormal blood clotting or low platelet count.

138. **What are the reasons for administration of medications to patients?**
   A. To treat acute illness or disease.
   B. As a part of the process of diagnosing illness, prevent illness, relief symptoms and to maintain general wellbeing.
   C. To provide relief from specific illness.
   D. All of the above.

139. **The nurse has made an error in documenting client care. Which appropriate action should the nurse take?**
   A. Draw a line through error, initial, date and document correct information.
   B. Document a late addendum to the nursing note in the client's chart.
   C. Tear the documented not out of the chart.
   D. Delete the error by using whiteout.

140. **A patient in your care is on regular oral morphine sulphate. As a qualified nurse, what legal checks do you need to carry out every time you administer morphine sulphate, which is in addition to those other drugs you would administer?**
A. Check to see whether the patient has become addicted.
B. Check the stock of oral morphine sulphate in the CD cupboard with another registered nurse and record this in the control drug book; then ask the patient to prove the identity to you.
C. Check the stock of oral morphine sulphate in the CD cupboard with another registered nurse and record this in the control drug book together, check the correct prescription and identity of the patient.
D. Check to see if the patient has become tolerant to the medication so it is no longer effective as analgesia

141. **In what quadrant should intramuscular injections be given into the buttocks?**
A. Upper innermost quadrant.
B. Upper outermost quadrant.
C. Lower innermost quadrant.
D. Lower outermost quadrant

142. **All should be seen in a good documentation except:**
A. Name and signature, position, date and time.
B. A correct, consistent and factual data.
C. Abbreviations, jargon, meaningless phrases and irrelevant subjective statements.
D. Legible handwriting.

143. **The nurse is caring for a patient who has a history of opioid abuse and is monitoring the client for signs of withdrawal symptoms. Which manifestations are specifically associated with withdrawal from opioids?**
   A. Depressed feelings, high drug, craving, fatigue and agitation.
   B. Dilated pupils, tachycardia, and diaphoresis.
   C. Tachycardia, hypertension, sweating and tremors.
   D. Yawning, irritability, diaphoresis, cramps and diarrhea

144. **Opioid toxicity are the following signs and symptoms except:**
   A. Constricted pupils.
   B. Decreased respiration.
   C. Drowsiness.
   D. Insomnia.

## Moving and Positioning

145. What serious condition is observed and noticed if a patient is placed in the Lloyd Davies position during surgery?
    A. Cardiac arrest
    B. Stroke
    C. Compartment syndrome
    D. There are no drawbacks to the Lloyd Davies position.

146. Your patient has bronchitis and has difficulty in clearing his chest. What position would help to maximize the drainage of secretions?
    A. Standing up and taking deep breathe
    B. Sitting up   leaning on pillows and inhaling humidified oxygen
    C. Lying in supine position while using nebulizer.
    D.  Lying in a lateral position and had humidified air.

147. How does the structures of the human body work together to provide support and assist in movement?
    A. The muscles provide a structural frame work, moving by contracting or extending, crossing at least one joint and attached to the articulating bones
    B. The muscles provide the structural frame work and are moved by bones to which they are attached by ligaments.
    C.  The skeleton provide the structural frame work, this is moved by ligaments that extend and contract.
    D. The skeleton provide a structural frame work, this is moved by the muscles that contract or extend and in order to function well it has to cross at least one joint which are attached to the articulating bones.

148. **A patient needs weighing, as he is due for a medication that is administered base on bodyweight. He experiences severe pain on movement so he is reluctant to move, particularly in attempt to stand up. What would you do?**
    A. Clearly document in the patients chart that the weight cannot be obtained.
    B. Offer the patient pain reliever and either use bed scales or a hoist with built in scales.
    C. Discuss the case with your colleagues and agree to guess his body weight until he agrees to stand and use the chair scales.
    D. Omit the drug as it is not safe to give it without his information; inform the doctor and document your actions.

149. **What should a patient not do on using a Zimmer frame?**
    A. It can be used outside.
    B. Don't carry any other thing with walker.
    C. Push walker forward when using it.
    D. Slide walker forward.

150. **What does 'muscle 'atrophy' mean?**
    A. Loss of muscle mass
    B. A change in the shape of muscles
    C. Disease of the muscle
    D. Accumulation of fluid in the muscle.

151. **A patient, who had stroke, sustained dysphagia. Which member of the interdisciplinary team should a nurse contact?**
    A. Physiotherapist.
    B. Speech therapist.
    C. Neurophysiologist.
    D. Dietician.

152. **While teaching a patient to walk in a Zimmer walker, which is the most appropriate advice?**
    A. Lift the walker 10 inches forward then take 2 steps and come in the middle.
    B. Slide the walker 10 inches forward then take small steps to maintain balance.
    C. Lift the walker 5 minutes forward then take 1 step and come in the middle.
    D. Slide walker 5 minutes backward and change with the leg.

153. **A nurse is teaching a patient about crutch walking which of the following is not correct?**
    A. Take long strides.
    B. Take small strides.
    C. Instruct to put weight on hands.
    D. Teach to step out the unhurt leg.

154. **The nurse is giving the client with a left cast crutch walking instructions using the three point gait. The client is allowed touchdown of the affected leg. The nurse tells the client to advance the:**
    A. Left leg and right crutch then right leg and left crutch.
    B. Crutches and then both legs simultaneously.
    C. Crutches and the right leg then advance the left leg.
    D. Crutches and the left leg then advance the right leg.

155. **Nurses are not using a hoist to transfer patient. They said it was not well maintained. What would you do?**
    A. Make a written report.
    B. Complain verbally.
    C. Take a picture for evidence.
    D. Do nothing.

156. **What is abduction?**
   A. Any motion of the limbs or other body parts that pulls away from midline of the body.
   B. The bending of a joint so as bring together the part it connects.
   C. The straightening of a joint.
   D. The movement of a body part toward the body's midline.

157. **What is the correct position for abdominal paracentesis**
   A. Lie the patient supine in bed with the head raised 45-50cm with a backrest
   B. Sitting upright at 45 to $60^0$
   C. Sitting upright at 60 to $75^0$
   D. Sitting upright at 75 to $90^0$

158. **When using crutches, what part of the body should absorb the patient's weight?**
   A. Armpits.
   B. Hands.
   C. Back.
   D. Shoulders.

159. **If your patients are unable to reposition themselves, how often should their position be changed?**
   A. 1 hourly.
   B. 2 hourly.
   C. 3 hourly.
   D. As often as possible.

160. Safe moving and handling of an anaesthetized patient is imperative to reduce harm to both the patient and staff. What is the minimum number of staff required to provide safe manual handling of a patient in the theatre?
    A. 1 each side, 1 at head.
    B. 2 each side, I at head.
    C. 1 each side, 1 at head, then 1 at feet.
    D. 2 each side, 1 at head, 1 at feet.

161. In what instance shouldn't you position a patient in a side-lying position?
    A. If they are pregnant
    B. If they have a spinal fracture
    C. If the pressure sore
    D. If they have lower limb pain.

162. Mr. John has had a cerebral vascular accident, so his left leg has increased tenderness, very stiff and difficult to position comfortably when he is in bed. What would you do?
    A. Give Mr. John analgesia and suggest he sleeps in the chair.
    B. Try to diminish increased tenderness by avoiding extra stimulation, ensuring his foot does not come into contact at the edge of the bed; support him with a pillow on his left leg, placed in a lateral position as well as keeping the knee flexed.
    C. Give Mr. John diazepam to reduce anxiety.
    D. Suggest a warm bath before he goes to bed. Then use pillows to support the stiff limb.

163. **When positioning the patient, supine in bed, why should you ensure that the patient is laid centrally in the bed?**
    A. To minimize the risk of injury to the practitioner.
    B. To ensure the airways is patent.
    C. To ensure patient comfort.
    D. To ensure the Spine and Limbs are aligned.

164. **Which of the following displays the proper use of zimmer frame?**
    A. Using a one point gait.
    B. Using a two point gait.
    C. Using a three point gait.
    D. Using a four point gait.

# Nutrition, Fluid Balance and Blood Transfusion

165. **What is the quantity of urine should an adult void in a day?**
    A. 800mls.
    B. 200 - 2000mls.
    C. 300 – 1500mls.
    D. 800 – 2000mls

166. **What type of diet would you recommend for your patient who has a newly formed stoma?**
    A. Encourage high-fiber foods to avoid constipation.
    B. Encourage lots of vegetable and fruits to avoid constipation.
    C. Encourage a varied diet as people can react differently.
    D. Avoid spicy foods because they can cause erratic function.

167. **People with blood group A are able to receive blood from the following?**
    A. Group A only
    B. Group AB or B
    C. Group A or O
    D. B or O

168. **How many cups of fluid do we need every day to keep us well hydrated?**
    A. 1 to 2 Cups.
    B. 2 to 4 Cups.
    C. 4 to 6 Cups.
    D. 6 to 8 Cups.

169. While brushing the teeth of a client the nurse observed that the client has bleeding gums. The nurse understands that the cause of this gingivitis is
A. Poor flossing.
B. Poor tarter removal.
C. Infection.
D. Lack of Vitamins.

170. Which condition is not a cause of diarrhea?
A. Ulcerative colitis.
B. Intestinal obstruction.
C. Hashimotos disease.
D. Food allergy.

171. Which among the following is a cause of Hemorrhoids?
A. High fiber rich diet.
B. Non-processed food.
C. Straining while passing stools.
D. Unsaturated fats in the diet.

172. A Jewish patient in a critical condition refuses the blood transfusion and states that his religion is against it. What should the nurse do?
A. Ignore client's wish and give him blood.
B. Tell the patient's relatives to take decision.
C. Accept the client's wish.
D. Force the client to give consent.

173. An overall risk of malnutrition of 2 or higher signifies
A. Low risk to malnutrition.
B. Medium risk of malnutrition.
C. High risk of malnutrition.
D. No risk.

174. **All are the symptoms of a patient in hypovolemic shock except.**
    *Choose several options*
    A. Bleeding.
    B. Diaphoresis.
    C. Cold clammy skin.
    D. Confusion.

175. **Protective diets are full of anti-oxidants and are helpful in diseased conditions, which of the following can be included in a protective diet?**
    A. Tomatoes, carrots and broccoli.
    B. Beef fish and chicken.
    C. Eggs dairy and cheese.
    D. Rice beans and pasta.

176. **In enteral feeding of a patient, how do you check the patency of the tube placement by:**
    A. Puling on the tube and then pushing it back in place.
    B. Testing for the PH of aspirate which should be less than 5.5.
    C. Infusing water or air and listening for bubbles.
    D. X-ray.

177. **A young mother who delivered 48hrs ago come back to the emergency department with post-partum hemorrhage. What type of PPH is it?**
    A. Primary post-partum hemorrhage.
    B. Secondary post-partum hemorrhage.
    C. Tertiary post-partum hemorrhage.
    D. Normal post-partum hemorrhage.

178. **A patient developed elevated temperature and pain in the loin during blood transfusion. This is indicative of:**
   A. Severe blood transfusion reaction.
   B. Common blood transfusion reaction.
   C. Adverse reaction.
   D. A minor irritability.

179. **A solution contain 12.5g of glucose in 0.25L. What is the percentage concentration (%) of this solution?**
   A. 5%
   B. 10%
   C. 25%
   D. 30%

180. **A litre bag of 5% glucose is prescribed over 4hours. If a standard giving set is used, at what rate should the drip be set?**
   A. 83.
   B. 60.
   C. 23
   D. 20.

181. **Patients with gastrointestinal bleeding may experience acute or chronic blood loss. Your patient is experiencing hematochezia. How would you recognize it?**
   A. Red or maroon-coloured stool rectally.
   B. Coffee ground emesis.
   C. Black, tarry stool.
   D. Vomiting of bright red or maroon blood.

182. On physical examination of a 15 year old female patient, you notice the posterior aspect of the knuckles of her hand. This is an indicative of:
    A. Self-induced vomiting and she likely has bulimia nervosa.
    B. A genetic disorder and her siblings should also be tested.
    C. Self-mutilation and correlates with anxiety.
    D. A connective tissue disorder and she should be referred to dermatology.

183. What do you need to monitor in other to avoid complications and to ensure optimal nutritional status in patients being fed through the means of enteral feeding
    A. Blood glucose levels, full blood count, stoma site and bodyweight.
    B. Eye sight, hearing, full blood count, and lung function and stoma site.
    C. Assess swallowing, patient choice, fluid balance, capillary refill time.
    D. Daily urinalysis, ECG, protein levels and arterial pressure.

184. The nurse monitors the serum electrolyte levels of a client who is taking digoxin (Lanoxin). Which of the following electrolyte imbalances is common cause of digoxin toxicity? *Choose several options.*
    A. Hypocalcemia.
    B. Hyponatremia.
    C. Hypomagnesemia.
    D. Hypokalemia.

185. A patient has been suffering from severe diarrhea and is showing signs of dehydration. Which of the following is not a classic symptom of dehydration?
    A. Passing small amount of urine frequently.
    B. Dizziness or light-headedness.

C. Dark-coloured urine.

D. Thirst.

186. **Dehydration is a particular concern in ill health. If a patient is receiving intravenous (IV) fluid replacement and is having their fluid balance recorded, which of the following statements is true of a client who is said to be in a 'positive fluid balance'?**

A. The fluid output has exceeded the input.

B. The doctor may consider increasing the IV drip rate.

C. The fluid balance chart can be stopped as 'positive' in this instance means 'good'.

D. The fluid input has exceeded the output.

187. **A patient had an abdominal surgery and will not be able to meet nutritional needs through oral intake. The patient was placed on enteral feeding. How would you position the patient when feeding is being administered?**

A. Sitting upright at 30 to $45^0$

B. Sitting upright at 45 to $60^0$

C. Sitting upright at 60 to $75^0$

D. Sitting upright at 75 to $90^0$

188. **A patient is admitted to the ward with symptoms of acute diarrhea. What should be your initial management?**

A. Assessment, protective isolation, universal precautions.

B. Assessment, source isolation, antibiotic therapy.

C. Assessment, protective isolation, ant motility medication.

D. Assessment, source isolation, universal precautions.

189. **The signs and symptoms of early fluid volume deficit are, except**

A. Decreased urine output.

B. Concentrated urine.

C. Decreased pulse rate.

D. Decreased skin turgor.

190. **A patient has Low BMI but she thought that she is fat. Whom do you refer her to?**
    A. Dietician.
    B. Mental health.
    C. Professional.
    D. Physiotherapists

191. **Which of the following is the most common aneurysm site?**
    A. Circle of Wills.
    B. Abdominal aorta.
    C. Renal arch.
    D. Hepatic artery.

192. **A patient has been admitted for nutritional support and started receiving a hyperosmolar feed yesterday. He presents with diarrhea and has no pyrexia. What is likely to be the cause?**
    A.    The feed.
    B. Food poisoning.
    C. An infection.
    D. Being in hospital.

193. **A patient has his intake to be 2437ml and output is 750ml, calculate the fluid volume balance.**
    A. 1197 (Negative Balance).
    B. 1687 (Negative Balance).
    C. 1687 (Positive Balance).
    D. 1197 (Positive Balance).

194. **What is the immediate treatment for severe bleeding?**
    A. Allow the wound to bleed and wash with soap and water.
    B. Place a sterile bandage or clean cloth and add pressure.
    C.  Clean the wound and plaster.
    D. Elevate the hand while the wound is still open.

195.    **Symptoms of dehydration are:**
   A. Increased pulse rate and BP
   B. Increased pulse rate and decreased BP
   C. Decreased pulse rate and increased BP
   D. Decreased skin turgor

196.    **These fruits can be recommended to a client with Crohn's disease except.**
   A. Papaya
   B. Mango.
   C. Cantaloupe.
   D. Strawberries.

197. **Mr. Matthew is receiving blood transfusion after a total hip replacement operation. Within 15 minutes of checking his vital signs he complained of fever and waste pain. What is the indication of this signs and symptoms?**
   A. Common adverse reaction.
   B. Renal Colic.
   C. Urinary infection
   D. Serious adverse reaction.

## Observation

198. You are caring for a patient who has had a recent head injury and you have been asked to carry out neurological observations every 15 minutes. You access and find out that his pupils are unequal and one is not reactive to light. You are no longer able to arouse him. What is your next action?

   A. Break down the patient Glasgow Coma Scale as follows: best verbal response V=XX, best motor response M=XX and eye opening E=XX. Use this when you hand over.
   B. This is a medical emergency. Basic airway, breathing, the circulation should be attended to urgently and help should be sought.
   C. Continue with your neurological assessment, calculate your Glasgow Coma Scale (GCS) and document clearly.
   D. Refer to the neurological team.

199. What are the key nursing observations needed for a patient receiving opioids frequently?

   A. Respiratory rate, bowel movement record and pain assessment and score.
   B. Checking the patient is not addicted by looking at their blood pressure.
   C. Lung function tests, oxygen saturation and addiction levels.
   D. Daily completion of a Bristol stool chart, urinalysis, and a record of the frequency with which the patient reports breakthrough pain.

200. A patient puts out his arm so that you can take his blood pressure. What type of consent is this?

   A. Verbal.
   B. Written.
   C. Implied.
   D. None of the above, consent is not required.

201. **The CQC describes compassion as what?**
    A. Intelligent kindness
    B. Smart confidence
    C. Creative commitment
    D. Gifted courage

202. **Which layer of the skin contains blood and lymph vessels and sebaceous glands?**
    A. Epidermis
    B. Dermis
    C. Subcutaneous layer
    D. All of the above.

203. **Holistic care involves: (*Choose several options*)**
    A. Physical Care
    B. Economic care
    C. Spiritual Care
    D. Social Care

204. **Compassionate care is described as:**
    A. Empathy
    B. Dignity
    C. Respect

205. **Immediately following Lumber Puncture to a client, she developed deterioration of consciousness, bradycardia, and increased systolic blood pressure. What is the result of the manifestation of these symptoms?**
    A. Normal reaction.
    B. Client has brain stem herniation.
    C. Spinal headache.
    D. Hyperflexia.

206. **The most common symptom of Type 1, Diabetes mellitus is**
    A. Thirst.
    B. Weight loss.
    C. Ketoacidosis.
    D. Diaphoresis.

207. **In the immediate post-operative period, what is the main priority?**
    A. Taking care of the airway.
    B. Watching for blood lose.
    E. Monitoring urine output.
    C. When septicaemia is suspected.
    D. Getting the consent.

208. **A patient is given penicillin tablet. After 12 hours the patient developed itching, rash and shortness of breath. What could be the reason?**
    A. Speed shock.
    B. Allergic reaction.
    C. Anaphylactic reaction.
    D. Bradycardia.

209. **A patient on Post-op was found crying, she said that the pain has not reduced even after given an analgesic. What is your next action as a nurse?**
    A. Call the doctor.
    B. Give a semi-reclined position to the patient.
    C. Give a heat pad for application.
    D. Provide a glass of water.

210. **Which is the most common sign of dehydration in older adults?**
    A. Reduced skin turgor.
    B. Bruises.
    C. Skin lesions.
    D. Pale/Cyanosis.

211. It is unsafe for a spinal tap to be undertaken if the patient: *Choose several options.*
    A. Has bacterial meningitis.
    B. Papilledema.
    C. Intracranial mass is suspected.
    D. Site skin infection.

212. You are monitoring a patient in the ICU when suddenly his consciousness drops and the size of one of his pupil becomes smaller what do you?
    A. Call the doctor.
    B. Refer to neurology team.
    C. Continue to monitor patient using GCS and record.
    D. Consider this as an emergency and prioritize ABC.

213. A patient is placed on observation and monitoring, hourly, when can the nurse formally document the findings?
    A. Every hour.
    B. When there are significant changes to the patient's condition.
    C. At the end of the shift.
    D. Everyday.

214. A patient is on Post Op liver biopsy, which of the following is a sign of intense complication?
    A. HR of 104, RR of 24, Temp of $37.5^{0c}$
    B. Nausea and vomiting.
    C. Pain.
    D. Bleeding.

215. **A patient is on post-operative repair of tibia and fibula, the possible signs of Compartment syndrome include?** *Choose several options.*
    A. Numbness and tingling.
    B. Cool dusky toes.
    C. Pain.
    D. Toes swelling.

216. **Common signs and symptoms of a hypoglycaemia exclude:**
    A. Feeling hungry.
    B. Sweating.
    C. Anxiety or irritability.
    D. Ketoacidosis.

217. **Which of the following is not a symptom of an ectopic pregnancy?**
    A. Pain.
    B. Bleeding.
    C. Vomiting.
    D. Diarrhoea.

218. **Orthostatic hypotension is diagnosed if the systolic blood pressure drops by how many mmHg?**
    A. 20.
    B. 25.
    C. 30.
    D. 35.

219. **What is compassion?**
    A. It means that individuals are responsible for their actions and maybe asked to justify them.
    B. It is intelligent kindness and is majorly on how people perceive their care.
    C. It means all those in caring roles must have the ability to understand an individual's health and social needs.
    D. It enables us to do the right thing for the people we care for.

220. A patient presented with a spinal cord injury. What is the most common cause of autonomic dysreflexia (a sudden rise in blood pressure)?
   A. Bowel obstruction.
   B. Fracture below the level of the spinal lesion.
   C. Pressure sore.
   D. Urinary obstruction.

221. What are the most common effects of inactivity?
   A. Pulmonary embolism, urinary tract infection and fear of people.
   B. Deep arterial thrombosis, respiratory infection, fear of movement, loss of consciousness, deconditioning of cardiovascular system leading to an increased risk of angina.
   C. Loss of weight, frustration and deep vein thrombosis.
   D. Depression and anxiety, social isolation, loss of independence, exacerbation of symptoms, rapid loss of strength in leg muscles, deconditioning of cardiovascular system leading to increased risk of chest infection, and pulmonary embolism.

222. How many phases of korotkoff sounds are there?
   A. 3.
   B. 4.
   C. 5.
   D. 6.

223. All are the symptoms of Impacted Earwax except.
   A. Dull hearing.
   B. Dizziness.
   C. Reflux cough.
   D. Sneezing.

224. **Accurate postoperative observations are key to assessing a patient's deterioration or recovery. The Modified Early Warnings Score (MEWS) is a scoring system that support aim. What is the primary purpose of MEWS?**
    A. Identifies patient at risk of deterioration.
    B. Improves communication between nursing staff and doctors.
    C. Accesses the impact of pre-existing conditions and postoperative recovery.
    D. Identifies potentials respiratory distress.

225. **All of the following subjective client data would be documented in the medical record by the nurse except?**
    A. Client's face is pale.
    B. Cervical lymph nodes are palpable.
    C. Nursing assistant reports client refused lunch.
    D. Client feel nauseated.

# Patient Comfort and End of Life Care

226.　　Which is not among reasons why most elderly people are prone to postural hypotension?
   A. Because of medications and conditions that cause hypovolemia.
   B. Because of activities and exercises.
   C. Because of a number of underlying problems with blood pressure control.
   D. Because of the baroreflex mechanisms which control heart rate and vascular conditions declines with age.

227. Your patient has undergone a formation of a loop colostomy. What important considerations should be borne in mind when selecting an appropriate stoma appliance for your patient?
   A. Dexterity of the patient, consistency of effluent, types of stoma.
   B. Patient preference, type of stoma, consistence of effluent, state of peristomal skin, dexterity of patient.
   C. Patient preference, lifestyle, position of stoma, consistency of effluent, state of peristomal skin, dexterity of patient, type of stoma.
   D. Cognitive ability, lifestyle, dexterity impairment, position of stoma, skin barrier, type of stoma, consistency of effluent, patient preference.

228. A patient is at the end stage of palliative care. Which among the following is not advisable?
   A. Giving analgesics and trying to relieve the symptoms.
   B. Talk to family and friends to provide a psychological support.
   C. Resuscitation.
   D. Make the patient sit outside and engage in the activities he likes.

**229.** **Who among the patients with these symptoms listed below are more prone to Coronary artery disease?**
    A. Hypotension, smoker, DM, obese women, non-sedentary lifestyle.
    B. Hypotension, smoker, DM, obese men with, non-sedentary lifestyle.
    C. Hypertension, smoker, obese men, sedentary lifestyle.
    D. Hypertension, obese women, diabetes, sedentary lifestyle.

**230.** **What are the symptoms of compensated shock?**
    A. Tachycardia, vasoconstriction and confusion.
    B. Bradycardia, low blood pressure and drowsy.
    C. Circulatory collapse, cardiovascular dysfunction, brain stem damage.
    D. Tachycardia, Circulatory collapse, low blood pressure.

**231. Compassion in practice, the culture of compassionate care encompasses**
    A. Care, Compassion, Competence, Communication, Courage, Commitment.
    B. Care, Compassion, Competence.
    C. Competence, Communication, Courage.
    D. Care, Courage, Commitment.

**232. The DVT TEDS stockings affect circulation by?**
    A. Increasing blood flow velocity in the legs by compression of the deep venous system.
    B. Decreasing blood flow velocity in legs compression of the deep venous system.
    C. Allow normal blood flow velocity in the legs.
    D. Prone position will enhance it.

**233.** **The conditions that causes orthostatic hypotension in the elderly are: *Choose several options.***
    A. Dehydration.
    B. Anemia
    C. Pharma therapeutic agents.
    D. Positional changes in blood pressure and heart rate.

234. **Which statement is not true about acute illness?**
    A. A disease with a rapid onset and/or a short course one.
    B. It will eventually resolve without any medical supervision.
    C. It is rapidly progressive and in need of urgent care.
    D. It is prolonged, do not resolve spontaneously, and is rarely captured completely.

235. **A patient is agitated and very anxious. She is also finding it difficult to sleep, reporting that she is in pain. What would you do at this point?**
    A. Tell her to score her pain level, describe its intensity, duration, the site and any relieving measures and what makes it worse, looking for nonverbal clues so that you can determine the appropriate method of pain management.
    B. Check the pain score, encourage her to take deep breathe, reposition her, after five (5) minutes, recheck the pain level. Give prescribed analgesic if pain is not relieved.
    C. Give her some sedatives to put her to sleep.
    D. Give her analgesic as prescribed. Also give her a warm milk to drink and reposition her pillows. Document actions.

236. **A client requested that he wants to go home against medical advice, what should you do?**
    A. Call the security guard.
    B. Allow the client to go home if he would not pose any threat to himself or others.
    C. Inform your supervisor or the physician.
    D. Inform the police.

**237. Nursing process is best illustrated as**
   A. Individualized approach to care.
   B. Patient with medical diagnosis.
   C. Task oriented care.
   D. All of the above.

**238. Which of the following is not a sign or symptom of speed shock?**
   A. Headache.
   B. A light feeling in the chest.
   C. Irregular pulse.
   D. Peripheral oedema.

**239. What does AVPU mean**
   A. Alert, verbalization, pain and unconsciousness.
   B. Alert, voice, pain and unresponsive
   C. Awake, voice, pain and unconsciousness
   D. Awake, verbalization, pain and unconsciousness

**240. What is primary care?**
   A. It is the Inital health care given by a health care provider in a community.
   B. GP practice, dental practice, community pharmacies and high street optometrists.
   C. It is a system of integrated care.
   D. It is a means of organizing work that is patient allocation.

**241. Aneurysm is mostly found in the elderly at which part of the body?**
   A. Vascular tissues.
   B. Hepatic vessels.
   C. Thoracic
   D. Abdominal.

242. **Why is pyrexia not evident in the elderly?**
    A. Due to lesser body fat.
    B. Due to aged hypothalamus.
    C. Due to immature T cells.
    D. Due to biologic changes.

243. **Which of the following senses fade last when a person dies?**
    A. Hearing
    B. Speaking
    C. Seeing
    D. Smelling

244. **Why are support stockings used?**
    A. To aid mobility.
    B. To promote arterial flow.
    C. To aid muscle.
    D. To promote venous flow.

245. **Who has the legal power to give permission for the body of a patient after death, to be donated for Research?**
    A. Directives by the patient himself before dying.
    B. The patient's family.
    C. The patient's GP.
    D. The medical Consultant in charge.

246. **.A patient asked an RN, "Can I tell you a secret?" What should be the RN's best response?**
    A. Yes because it develops trust which is central to the nursing practice.
    B. Yes and will share it with the relevant medical team.
    C. Yes I will share it with all the medical professionals who are supposed to know the secret.
    D. Yes I will keep the secret because it is confidential.

## Patient Safety

247. **What would you do if a patient with diabetes and peripheral neuropathy requires your assistance in cutting his toe nails?**
    A. Document clearly the reason for not cutting his toe nails and refer him to a chiropodist.
    B. Document clearly the reason for not cutting his nails and ask the ward sister to do it.
    C. Go ahead and do that and if you run into trouble, stop and refer to the chiropodist.
    D. Speak to the patient's GP to ask for referral to the chiropodist, but make a start while the patient is in hospital.

248. **Clara has just returned from theatre following surgery on her left arm. She has a PCA infusion connected on admission. On assessment there is poor control over her right hand and in severe pain. What would you do?**
    A. Contact the pain management team, anesthetist to discuss the situation on how to relieve this condition.
    B. Educate her family to push the button when the patient ask for it and encourage them to tell the nursing staff when the leave the ward so that the nurse can take over her care.
    C. The patient should have prescribed paracetamol.
    D. Routinely offer the patient an IM and document clearly.

249. **A patient in your care hit his head on the bedside locker when reaching down to pick up something but fell. What do you do?**

   A.    Let the patient's relatives know so that they don't make a complaint and write an incident report for yourself so you remember the details in case there are problems in the future.

   B. Help the patient to sit in a comfortable position, commence neurological observations and ask the patients doctor to come and review them, checking the injury isn't serious. When this has taken place, write up what happened and any future care in the nursing notes.

   C. Discuss the incident with the nurse in charge, and contact your union representative in case you get into trouble.

   D. Help the patient to a safe comfortable position, observe for any injury and report the incident to the nurse in charge, call a doctor. Complete an incident form. At an appropriate time, discuss the incident with the patient and, if they wish, their relatives.

250. **The nurse discloses a patient's information to a third party when:**
   A. It is by the law/ order.
   B. It is justified for public interest.
   C. The media insists for disclosure.
   D. It is by law/ order and justified for public interest.

251. **While having lunch at the cafeteria, your colleague suddenly collapsed. What is your next action?** *Choose more than one options.*
   A. Assess the environment and remove any danger.
   B. Assess for the level of consciousness.
   C. Call for help
   D. No actions should be done now since you're on lunch.

252. **What is the best way to prevent a patient who is receiving an enteral feed from aspirating?**
    A. Put them on supine position.
    B. Place in low fowler's position of 45° angle.
    C. Put them on a lateral position.
    D. Monitor the oxygen level regularly.

253. **A nurse documented an intervention on a wrong patient chart. What are the necessary actions you should take care of in other to maintain patient safety and have a continuity of care?**
    A. Cross the wrong entry with a line. Indicating cancellation. Write the date, time, name and signature, document the care given correctly.
    B. Discard the paper or document.
    C. Do not alter patient's record.
    D. Inform the nurse manager, let her do the correct entry and sign.

254. **Early ambulation prevents all complications except:**
    A. Chest infection and lung collapse.
    B. Muscle wasting.
    C. Thrombosis.
    D. Surgical site infection.

255. **Patient-centered care is best defined as:**
    A. The care that is focused on the environment.
    B. The care which is focused on the health care team.
    C. The care that is focused on the patient.
    D. The care focused on the doctor.

256. Which of the following population group is at risk of developing cardiovascular disease? *Choose several options.*
   A.  Male, female, obese, diabetic, hypertensive, sedentary lifestyle.
   B.  Female, forty years, fertile or on reproductive age.
   C.  Smoker, diabetic and alcoholic.
   D.  Male, drug abuse, hypertensive

257. A patient wants to leave hospital against medical advice. The doctors are concerned about the patient's competent under the mental capacity act. What should the nurse do next? *Choose several options.*
   A.  Let the patient go, if he is competent and in his full sense.
   B.  Call for police.
   C.  If he does not have the mental capacity, restrain the patient and treat.
   D.  Call the security and make the patient stay until the doctor complete their assessment.

258. If you witness or suspect there is an immediate risk at hand for the safety of people in your care what should you do? *Choose several Options.*
   A.  Report your concerns immediately, in writing to the appropriate person or body escalating concerns to the NMC.
   B.  Report the event to the NMC.
   C.  Ask for advice from your professional body if unsure on what actions to take.
   D.  Protect client confidentiality.

## Pre-operative Care

**259. What is meant by 'Gillick competent'?**

    A. Children under the age of 12 who are believed to have enough intelligence, competence and understanding to fully appreciate what's involved in their treatment.

    B. Children under the age of 16 who are believed to have enough intelligence, competence and understanding to fully appreciate what is involved in their treatment and give consent without the need for parental permission.

    C. Children under the age of 18 who are believed to have enough intelligence, competence and understanding to fully appreciate what is involved in their treatment.

    D. Children under the lawful age of consent who are believed not to have enough intelligence, competence and understanding to fully appreciate what's involved in the treatment.

**260. What are the required step(s) in Informed consent prior to surgery?**

    A. Get the patient's understanding of the procedure by letting them know the benefits, probably complications stated by the Physicians and then they signed the consent that they were well informed.

    B. Tell the patient about the surgery and give him consent form to sign.

    C. Get the patient's understanding of the procedure by letting him know the benefit, complications and then signed that he was well informed.

    D. Explain the details from his admission, about the surgery and discharge.

261. An adult has been administered pre- operative medication for his surgery. As the nurse was going through the client's chat, she realized that the consent form has not been signed. Which of the following is the best action for the nurse to do?
    A. Assume it is emergency surgery and consent is implied.
    B. Get the consent form and have the client sign it.
    C. Tell the physician that the consent form is not signed.
    D. Have a family member sign the consent form.

262. A patient is scheduled to undergo an Elective Surgery. What is the last thing that should be done?
    A. Assess/Obtain the patient's understanding, the consent to the procedure, and participate in the decision making process.
    B. Ensure pre-operative NPO, the prescribed pain reliever, and expected procedure are carried out and discussed.
    C. Discuss the risk involved, complications and prognosis.
    D. To document the details of the procedure in the anesthetic record.

263. You were administering a pre-operative medication to a patient via IM route. Suddenly you developed a needle-stick injury. Which of the following interventions will not be appropriate for you to do?
    A. Prevent the wound from bleeding.
    B. Wash the wound using running water and plenty of soap.
    C. Do not suck the wound.
    D. Dry the wound and cover it with waterproof plaster or dressing.

264. **Your patient has a bulky oesophageal tumour and is waiting for surgery. When he tries to eat, food gets stuck and gives him heartburn. What is the most likely route that will be chosen to provide him with the nutritional support he needs?**
    A. Nasogastric tube feeding.
    B. Feeding via a percutaneous endoscopic gastrostomy (PEG).
    C. Feeding through a radiological inserted gastrostomy (RIG).
    D. Continue oral food.

265. **Who should mark the skin with indelible pen before the surgery?**
    A. The surgeon
    B. The Anesthetist nurse.
    C. The Anesthetist doctor.
    D. The patient should indicate where it should be done.

266. **Why is it important that patients are required to stop eating at least 6 hours before surgery?**
    A. To prevent vomiting and chest infections.
    B. To empty the stomach.
    C. In other for them to sleep well
    D. To reduce the risk of aspirations, reflux and inhalation of gastric contents.

# Psychosocial Care

267. After two weeks of receiving lithium therapy, a patient in the psychiatric unit becomes depressed. Which of the following evaluations of the patient's behaviour by the nurse would be most accurate?
    A. The treatment plan is not effective; the patient requires a larger dose of lithium.
    B. This is a normal response to lithium therapy; the patient should continue with the current treatment plan.
    C. This is a normal response to lithium therapy; the patient should be monitored for suicidal behaviour.
    D. The treatment plan is not effective; the patient requires an antidepressant.

268. A seventeen (17) year old patient had recently undergone an orthopedic surgery due to a road traffic accident. He is stable and can take care of himself. Few days later he was withdrawn and could not attempt his personal care anymore even though his condition seem stable. What could be the reason for this behavior?
    A. He wants to repress his feelings to forget the accident.
    B. He is depressed and he has gone to his earlier state of dependency. He wants the same attention he had received when he was ill.
    C. He is depressed.
    D. He wants to displace his experience by not taking care of himself.

269. Which of the following is not a usual sign and symptom associated with depression
    A. Anorexia.
    B. Feeling of sadness and hopelessness.
    C. Increased energy.
    D. Reserved and isolated.

270. A client was admitted at the psychiatric unit to be monitored for depression and suicidal behavior. On the 3rd day he seems to be very happy and is interacting with others, what could be this symptom concluded to be?
    A. He has finalized his plan for suicide.
    B. He's improving.
    C. He has made new friends.
    D. He is contemplating of committing suicide.

271. A 19 years old patient who was involved in an accident is observed not eating the meals that she previously ordered and refused to take her bath even when she was already in a recovery stage. As a nurse what do you think is the best explanation for her reaction to the accident that happened to her?
    A. Suppression.
    B. Repression.
    C. Regression.
    D. Undoing.

272. You believe that an adult you know and supported has been a victim of physical abuse which might be considered criminal. What should you do to support the police in the investigation?
    A. Question the adult thoroughly to get as much information as possible.
    B. Take photographs of any signs of abuse or other potential evidence before cleaning up the victim or the crime scene.
    C. Explain to the victim that you cannot speak to them unless a police officer is present.
    D. Make an accurate record of what the person has said to you.

**273. What is the difference between denial & collusion?**

    A. Denial is when a healthcare professional refuses to tell a patient their diagnosis for the protection of the patient whereas collusion is when healthcare professionals & the patient agree on the information to be told to relatives & friends.

    B. Denial is when a patient refuses treatment & collusion is when a patient agrees to it.

    C. Denial is a coping mechanism used by an individual with the intention of protecting themselves from painful or distressing information whereas collusion is withholding information from the patient with the intention of protecting them.

    D. Denial is a normal acceptable response by a patient to a life-threatening diagnosis whereas collusion is not.

**274. If you were explaining anxiety to a patient, what would be the main points to include?**

    A. Signs of anxiety include behaviours such as muscle tension. Palpitations, a dry mouth, fast shallow breathing, dizziness & an increased need to urinate or defecate.

    B. Anxiety has three aspects: Physically, bodily sensations related to flight & fight response; behaviourally, such as avoiding the situation, and cognitive (thinking), such as imagining the worst to happen.

    C. Anxiety is all in the mind, if they learn to think differently, it will go away.

    D. Anxiety has three aspects: Physical – such as running away, behavioural – such as imagining the worse (catastrophizing), & cognitive (thinking) – such as needing to urinate.

275. A 52-year old man was admitted to a hospital after sustaining a severe head injury in an automobile accident. When the patient died, the nurse observed that the patient's wife was comforting other family members. Which of the following interpretations of this behaviour is most justifiable?
   A. She has already moved through the stages of the grieving process.
   B. She is repressing anger related to her husband's death.
   C. She is experiencing shock and disbelief related to her husband's death.
   D. She is demonstrating resolution of her husband's death.

276. A patient with a history of schizophrenia is admitted to the acute psychiatric care unit. He muttered to himself as the nurse attempts to take a history and yelled, 'I don't want to answer any more questions! There are too many voices in this room!" Which of the following assessment questions should the nurse ask next?
   A. "Are the voices telling you to do things?
   B. "Do you feel as though you want to harm yourself or anyone else"?
   C. Who else is talking in this room? It's just you and me. "I don't hear any other voices".
   D. Can you tell me about it? "What do you hear about this voices"?

277. The nurse cares for a client diagnosed with conversion reaction. The nurse identifies the client is utilizing which of the following defense mechanisms?
   A.   Introjection.
   B.   Displacement.
   C.   Identification
   D.   Repression.

# Respiratory Care

**278. All are risk factors of Coronary artery disease except:**
   A. Obesity.
   B. Smoking.
   C. High blood pressure.
   D. Gender.

**279. In which of the following situation might nitrous oxide (Entonox) be considered?**
   A. A wound dressing change for short- term pain relief or the removal of a chest drain for reduction of anxiety.
   B. Turning a patient who has bowel obstruction because there is an expectation that they may have pain from pathological fractures.
   C. For pain relief during the insertion of a chest drain for the treatment of pneumothorax.
   D. For pain relief during a wound dressing for a patient who has had a radical head and neck cancer that involved the jaw.

**280.** **You are looking after an emaciated 80 year-old man who has been admitted to your ward with acute exacerbation of chronic obstructive airways disease (COPD). He is currently so short of breath that it is difficult for him to move. What are some of the actions you would take to prevent him developing a pressure ulcer?**

A. He will be at high risk of developing a pressure ulcer, so place him on a pressure relieving mattress.

B. Assess his risk of developing a pressure ulcer with a risk assessment tool. If indicated, admit to an appropriate pressure-relieving mattress and cushion as his bed and chair respectively. Reassess the patient's pressure areas at least twice a day and keep them clean and dry. Review his fluid and nutritional intake and support him to make changes as indicated.

C. Assess his risk of developing a pressure ulcer with a risk assessment tool and reassess every week. Reduce his fluid intake to avoid him becoming incontinent and making the pressure areas to become damp with urine.

D. He is at high risk of developing a pressure ulcer because of his recent acute illness, poor nutritional intake and reduced mobility. By giving him his prescribed antibiotics therapy and referring him to the dietician and physiotherapist will reduce the risk.

281. You are caring for a patient with a history of COAD who is requiring 70% humidified oxygen via a facemask. You are monitoring his response to therapy by observing his colour, degree of respiration distress and respiratory rate. The patient's oxygen saturations have been between 95% and 98% in addition, the doctor has been taking arterial blood gas. What is the reason for this?

    A. Oximeters may be unreliable under certain circumstances, e.g. if tissue perfusion is poor, if the environment is cold and if the patient nails are covered with nail polish.

    B. Arterial blood gas shows the level of Oxygen in the blood and this is part of the patient's care.

    C. Pulse oximeters provide excellent evidence of oxygenation, but they do not measure the adequacy of ventilation.

    D. Arterial blood gas measures both oxygen and carbon dioxide levels and therefore gives an indication of both ventilation and oxygenation.

282. A patient with Lung cancer suffers from breathlessness, which should be the worst possible measure to take as a treatment?

    A. Crystal therapy by Traditional therapist.

    B. Educating to control the breath by chest Physiotherapist.

    C. Chest physiotherapy, by Physiotherapist.

    D. Maintain the chest tube drainage system.

283. What is the common cause of Airway obstruction in an unconscious patient?

    A. Oropharyngeal tumour.

    B. Laryngeal cyst.

    C. Obstruction of foreign body.

    D. Tongue falling back.

284. A patient has been discharged with continuing Oxygen therapy, 2 Litres, through the Nasal cannula. When you visited the patient you found out that the patient is dyspnoeic, anxious and frightened. What is the best action for the nurse to take?
    A. Administer tab. Or morph which is prescribed as PNO.
    B. Try to calm down the patient.
    C. Decrease the level of Oxygen.
    D. Increase the level of Oxygen.

285. A patient with COPD is discharged from the hospital, what advice should the nurse give to prevent exacerbation of the condition?
    A. Advise the patient to take measures to quit smoking.
    B. Advise the patient to do breathing exercise.
    C. Teach purse lip breathing.
    D. Advise to maintain adequate hydration.

286. If an Oro-pharyngeal airway is inserted properly, what is the sign?
    A. Airway obstruction.
    B. Retching and vomiting.
    C. Bradycardia.
    D. Tachycardia.

287. In a COPD patients, what are the typical symptoms to observe?
    A. $CO_2$ high, $PO_2$ low.
    B. $CO_2$ low, $PO_2$ high.
    C. $CO_2$ low, $PO_2$ low.
    D. $CO_2$ high, $PO_2$ high.

288. **A terminally ill patient tells the nurse that he doesn't want CPR. What should the nurse do?**
    A. Force the patient to have the CPR that it is very important.
    B. Ask the relatives to talk to the patient.
    C. Tell the patient that his decision is absolutely right.
    D. Explain to him about advanced directives.

289. **A patient who is to receive Oxygen therapy needs?**
    A. A prescription requiring, the route, method and duration.
    B. No prescription is required unless he will use it at home.
    C. Prescription not required for oxygen therapy.
    D. A prescription but can be administered at any time.

290. **Normal heart rate for 1 to 2 years old?**
    A. 70- 110 beats per minute.
    B. 80 -140 beats per minute.
    C. 75 – 115 beats per minute.
    D. 60 – 150 beats per minute.

291. **Which of the following is an indication for Intra pleural chest drain insertion?**
    A. Pneumothorax.
    B. Tuberculosis.
    C. Asthma.
    D. Malignancy of the lungs.

292. **As a registered nurse in a unit what would you consider as priority for immediate care to a patient post operatively?**
    A. Pain relief.
    B. Blood loss.
    C. Airway patency.
    D. The effect of anesthetic.

**293. A patient experienced sensation of fluttering in his chest, light headedness, & chest pain. The doctor diagnosed atrial fibrillation. What is atrial fibrillation?**
    A. A rare, rapid and disorganized rhythm of heartbeats that rapidly leads to loss of consciousness and sudden death if not treated immediately.
    B. Episodes of abnormally fast heart rate at rest.
    C. The heart beats more slowly than normal and can cause people to collapse.
    D. A heart condition that causes an irregular and often abnormally fast heart rate.

**294. Which are the symptoms presented in anaphylactic shock?**
    A. Dizziness, Headache, feeling of impending doom.
    B. Dyspnea, wheezing, stridor, tachypnea.
    C. Hypotension, tachycardia, dysrhythmias.
    D. All of the above.

**295. If a patient is prescribed nebulizers, what is the minimum flow rate in litres per minute required?**
    A. 2 – 4 Litres.
    B. 4 – 6 Litres.
    C. 6 – 8 Litres.
    D. 8 – 10 Litres.

**296. In normal breathing, what is the main muscle (s) involved in inspiration?**
    A. The diaphragm.
    B. The lungs.
    C. The intercostal.
    D. All of the above.

297. **What percentage of the air we breathe is made up of oxygen?**
    A. 16%.
    B. 21%.
    C. 26%.
    D. 31%.

298. **A patient had collapse with an anaphylactic reaction. What symptoms would you expect to see?**
    A. The patient will experience a sense of impending doom, hyperventilate and be itchy all over.
    B. The patient will have a low blood pressure (hypotensive) and will have a fast heart rate (tachycardia) usually associated with skin and mucosal changes.
    C. The patient will quickly find breathing very difficult because of compromise to their airway or circulation.
    D. The patient will have a high blood pressure (hypertensive) and will have a fast heart rate.

299. **What is the most accurate method of calculating a respiratory rate?**
    A. Counting the number of respiratory cycles in 15 seconds and multiplying it by 4.
    B. Counting the number of respiratory cycles in 1 minutes. One cycle is equal to the complete rise and fall of the patient's chest.
    C. Not telling the patient, as this may make them conscious of their breathing pattern and influences the accuracy of the rate.
    D. Placing your hand on the patient chest and counting the number of respiratory cycles in 30 seconds and multiplying by 2.

**300. The correct management of an adult patient in Ventricular Fibrillation (VF) with cardiac arrest includes:**
   A. An initial shock with a manual defibrillator or when prompted by an Automated External Defibrillator (AED).
   B. Adenosine 500mcg IV.
   C. Adrenaline 1mg IV before first shock.
   D. Atropin.

**301. Respiratory protective equipment include:**
   A. Apron.
   B. Mask.
   C. Glove.
   D. Paper towels.

**302. A patient is in immediate recovery post-surgery. What should you monitor?**
   A. Breathing.
   B. Temperature.
   C. Blood loss.
   D. Pain.

**303. A patient in your ward complained that his heart is racing and the nurse found that his pulse was too fast when manually palpated. What should be the immediate action by the nurse?**
   A. Calm the patient and check his blood pressure and fluid balance.
   B. Check baseline observations and refer to the cardiologist's team.
   C. Shout for help.
   D. Assess and carry out a full set of observations: blood pressure, respiration rate, oxygen saturation and temperature rhythm, perform a 12 lead ECG. Call the attention of his Physician.

# Vulnerable Adults and Children

**304. What is an intermediate care home?**
- A. It is the day-to-day health care given by a health care provider.
- B. It includes a range of short-term treatment or rehabilitative services designed to promote independences.
- C. It is a system of integrated care.
- D. It is a means of organizing work that is patient allocation.

**305. You are assisting a doctor who is trying to assess and collect information from a child who does not seem to understand all that the doctor is telling and is restless. What will be your best response?**
- A. Stay quiet and remain with the doctor.
- B. Interrupt the doctor and ask the child the question.
- C. Remain with the doctor and try to gain confidence of the child and politely assess the child's level of understanding and help the doctor with the information he is looking for.
- D. Make the child quiet and ask his mother to stay with him.

**306. How can patients who need assistance at meal times be identified?**
- A. A red sticker.
- B. A color serviette.
- C. A red tray.
- D. Any of the above.

307. **A nurse assistant was found abusing an elderly patient verbally, what will be your action as a registered nurse?**
    A. Intervene immediately by halting the staff, make sure that the patient is safe and report to the authority.
    B. Ignore the situation.
    C. Report in the authority.
    D. Enquire about the incident with the patient later.

308. **Mr. Smith, an elderly patient with dementia wishes to go out of the hospital. What will be your appropriate action?**
    A. Allow him to leave, he is stable and not at risk of anything.
    B. Encourage the patient to stay and rather let his reasons for going out be known.
    C. Call the Police.
    D. Restraint him.

309. **In a Community setting, an elderly patient reported to you that he gave shopping money to his neighbor but he failed to bring groceries to him most times. What is your best response on this situation?**
    A. Tell the patient to report his neighbor to the police.
    B. Confront the neighbor regarding this complaint.
    C. Raise a concern and complete a safeguarding form and intervene.
    D. Ignore, maybe he is very old and does not think clearly.

310. **Safeguarding is the responsibility of:**
    A. Healthcare assistants.
    B. Registered nurses.
    C. Doctors.
    D. All of the above.

**311.** _____ is a behavioural risk factor when assessing the potential risks of falling in an older person.
A. Urination.
B. Meditation.
C. Poor nutrition and or fluid intake.
D. Lying down.

## Wound Management

312.    The phases of management of the burn injury are the following except:
A. Resuscitation/Emergent phase.
B. Restorative phase.
C. Acute phase.
D. Rehabilitative phase.

313.    Initial signs of phlebitis is
A. Hot and tender skin.
B. Signs of shock.
C. Cold skin with cyanosed nail bed.
D. Bleeding.

314.    When does the proliferation phase start in wound healing?
A. 10-24 days.
B. Within minutes.
C. 1-2 days.
D. 25 days or more.

315.    You have just finished dressing a wound of a patient with leg ulcer and you observed that the patient was depressed and withdrawn. You asked the patient if everything was okay. She said "yes". What is your next action?
A. Say "I observe you don't seem as usual. Are you sure you are okay?"
B. Say "Cheer up, shall I make a cup of tea for you?"
C. Accept her response and leave to attend to other patients.
D. Inform the doctor about the change of behavior.

316. **Wound care management plan should be done with what type of wound?**
    A. Complex wound.
    B. Simple wound.
    C. Infected wound.
    D. Any type of wound.

317. **Proper dressing for wound care should be?**
    A. High humidity, non-permeable, conformable, absorbent.
    B. Non-permeable, absorbent, low humidity, non-conformable.
    C. Conformable, low humidity, permeable, absorbent.
    D. Absorbent, permeable, high humidity, conformable.

318. **What do expect to assess in a grade 3 pressure ulcer?**
    A. Blistered wound on the skin.
    B. Open wound showing tissue.
    C. Open wound exposing muscles.
    D. Open wound exposing bones.

319. **A new, postsurgical wound is assessed by the nurse and is found to be hot, tender and swollen. How best would you describe it?**
    A. In the inflammation phase of healing.
    B. In the haemostasis phase of healing.
    C. In the reconstructive phase of wound healing.
    D. As an infected wound.

320. **How long does the 'inflammatory phase' of wound healing typically last?**
    A. 24hours.
    B. 3 to 24 days.
    C. 1 to 5 days.
    D. Just few minutes.

321. **Black wound are treated with debridement. Which type of debridement is most selective and least damaging?**
    A. Debridement with scissors.
    B. Debridement with wet to dry dressings.
    C. Mechanical debridement.
    D. Chemical debridement.

322. **A client's wound is draining thick yellow material. The nurse correctly describes the drainage as:**
    A. Sanguineous.
    B. Serous-sanguineous.
    C. Serous.
    D. Purulent.

323. **The nurse cares for a client with a wound in the late regeneration phase of tissue repair. The wound may be protected by applying:**
    A. Transparent film.
    B. Hydrogel dressing.
    C. Collagenase dressing.
    D. Wet to dry dressing.

324. **In what order should the four phases of wound healing be?**
    A. Inflammation, Proliferation, hemostasis, maturation.
    B. Hemostasis, Inflammation, Proliferation, maturation.
    C. Proliferation, hemostasis, maturation, inflammation.
    D. Maturation, inflammation, proliferation, hemostasis.

325. **A client has a diabetic ulcer on the lower leg. The nurse uses a hydrocolloid dressing to cover it. The procedure for application includes:**
    A. Cleaning the skin and wound with betadine.
    B. Removing all traces of residues for the old dressing.
    C. Choosing a dressing no more than quarter-inch larger than the wound size.
    D. Holding in place the hydrocolloid dressing for one minute to allow it to adhere.

326. A client is admitted to the Emergency Department after a motorcycle accident that resulted in the client's skidding across a cement parking lot. Since the client was wearing shorts, there are large areas on the legs where the skin is ripped off. This wound is best described as:
   A. Abrasion.
   B. Scar.
   C. Laceration.
   D. Eschar.

327. When would it be beneficial to use a wound care plan?
   A. In all chronic wounds.
   B. In all complex wounds.
   C. In all infected wounds.
   D. On every wound.

328. Which of the following method of wound closure is most suitable for a good cosmetic result following surgery?
   A. Skin clips.
   B. Tissue adhesive.
   C. Interrupted suture.
   D. Adhesive skin closure strips.

329. Which one of the follow types of wound is NOT suitable for negative pressure wound therapy?
   A. Partial thickness burns.
   B. Contaminated wounds.
   C. Diabetic and neuropathic ulcers.
   D. Traumatic wounds.

330. These are types of ideal wound dressing except which one?
   A. Low humidity
   B. Absorbent.
   C. Cost effective.
   D. The presence of gaseous exchange.

# NMC CBT Practice Test Answers.

## Assessment and Discharge Planning.

1. **B** "I should increase the fiber in my diet".
2. **A**. Maximize dependent living.
3. **C**. Speech Therapist.
4. **A**. within 24hours of admission
5. **B**. Understanding.
6. **A**. Foot/Ankle.
7. **A**. Understand information about the decision and remember that information.
   **B.** Use that information to make a decision.
   **C**. Communicate their decision by talking, using sign language or by any other means.
8. **B**. Deficiency of Insulin, **C**. Infection, **D**. Stress.
9. **C**. Assessment for the level of consciousness.
10. **A**. Rebound tenderness and guarding.
11. **D**. Epigastric pains worsens after eating and weight loss.
12. **B**. Temperature of $38.5^0C$, shivering tachycardia and hypertensive.
13. **C**. Observe the patient's breathing for ease and comfort, rate and pattern.
14. **C.** The patient has spiked in temperature, has a raised white blood cell (WBC), and in a confused state and the urine in their catheter bag is cloudy.
15. **A**. Blood and mucous in the faeces.
    **B**. Fatigue.
    **C**. Loss of appetite.
    **D**. Diarrhea.
16. **D**. All of the above
17. **C**. It is a form of documentation.
18. **D**. Alternating pressure.

19. **A**. That the patient can independently manage their stoma, and can get supplies.
20. **A**. Assessment
21. **B**. Intestinal obstruction.


## Communication
22. **D**. 7%
23. **A**. Squarely, open posture, leaning slightly forward, eye contact, relaxed.
24. **A**. Effective communication skill, mutual respect, constructive feedback and conflict management.
25. **D**. All of the above.
26. **B**. Communication and team work.
27. **D**. I'm sorry, your mother passed away.
28. **A**. Accept their wishes under Western Foods and Cultural differences considerations.
29. **A**. Dysphasia.
30. **A**. It becomes a threat to the public and when it is ordered by the court.
31. **D**. All of the above.
32. **A**. Listening, clarifying the concerns and feelings of the patient using open questions.
33. **D**. Tone.
34. **A**. Use shot statements and closed questions in a well-lit, quiet and familiar environment.
35. **C**. Relying on their family or friends to explain what you mean.
36. **B**. When you said you are hurt, what do you mean?
37. **B**. The course of the present illness.
38. **A**. Developmental level.
39. **A**. Introduction.
40. **C**. Tell the patient you are interested in what concerns them & that you are available to listen and keep it confidential.
41. **A**. Compassion, support & reassurance to the client.
42. **A**. Accepting.

## Infection Prevention and Control.

43. **B**. Shivering, 38.4°c, tachycardia and hypertensive.
44. **B**. Ask her to come and visit after 48hrs of recovery from the symptoms.
45. **B**. Take in the red plastic bag that disintegrates in high temperature.
46. **D**. Colitis.
47. **B**. Tuberculosis.
    **C**. Whooping cough.
48. **A**. Stoma or catheter bags.
49. **D**. None of the above.
50. **C**. Before and immediately after contact with patients, body fluids, mucous membranes and non-intact skin.
51. **C**. Nurse the patient in isolation, ensure that you wear appropriate personal protective equipment (PPE) and adhere to strict hand hygiene, for the purpose of preventing the spread of organisms from that patient to others.
52. **B**. Gently make the wound bleed, place under running water and wash thoroughly with soap and water. Cover any wound with a waterproof dressing to prevent entry of any other foreign material. Complete an incident form and inform your manager. Co-operate with any action to screen yourself or the patient for infection with blood borne virus but do not obtain blood or consent for testing from the patient yourself; this should be done by someone not involved in the incident.
53. **D**. Methicillin Resistant Staphylococcus Aureus.
54. **B**. The actions that should be taken in every care situation to protect patients and others from infection, regardless of what is known of the patient's status in regard to infection.
55. **B**. Client with a Central venous catheter (CVC).
56. **C**. Creutzfeldt- jakob.
57. **C**. Yellow and black stripe.
58. **D**. All of the above.
59. **C**. Disposal of waste.

# Laboratory Diagnostics and Tests.

60. **A**. Fever, diarrhea, anorexia, anemia, weight loss, colicky pains after eating, dehydration, electrolytes imbalance and malnutrition.
61. **C**. Atrial fibrillation.
62. **A**. Inadvertent puncture of pleural, a blood vessel or bile duct.
63. **B**. International Normalized Ratio.
64. **A**. Eat fluid based food or low residue diet and or drink more of fluid to avoid dehydration as soon as sedation has worn out.
65. **C**. For patients with increased ICP.
66. **C**. Collect at least 10mL of blood.
67. **C**. MRI.
68. **D**. Inoculate the aerobic culture first.
69. **D**. If peripheral circulation is impaired, collection of capillary blood is not advised, as the result might not be a true reflection of the physiological blood glucose level.
70. **A**. Gastroscopy.
71. **A**. A tool to evaluate the effectiveness of interventions and to know what needs to be improved.
72. **B**. One size fits all.
73. **C**. Conceptual and interpersonal skills.
74. **D.** Incentives to promote loyalty and performance.
75. **D**. Functional method.
76. **B**. Mental capacity act (2005).
77. **B**. Train these managers for them to focus on maintaining standards of care.
78. **A**. Anger.
79. **A**. Rehabilitation, Physiotherapy, Psychiatry, Acute care.
80. **D**. Talk to her privately and let her be aware that such behavior is not expected of nurses.
81. **D**. Raise the complaint in the incident report form and investigate the matter as well as inform the concerned authorities.

82. **D**. Counsel the patient to stay back in the hospital for him to get much better.
83. **C**. It helps to identify areas of improvement in the system pertaining to Nursing and medical practitioner.
    **D**. It helps to understand medical outcomes and the process only.
84. **D**. None of the above.
85. **D**. When there is no friend and family present to make a wish or take a decision for the client.
86. **C**. Practice effectively.
87. **B**. Only under close and direct supervision.
88. **C**. It ascertain in detail in nurses or clinical expertise.
89. **A**. 35 units.
90. **B**. Ask from your manager if there are qualified staff from the previous shift that can make up the number for your shift while you try to replace with new nurses to cover up.
91. **C**. Immediate nurse manager.
92. **D**. All of the above.
93. **A**. It means that individuals are responsible for their actions and may be asked to justify them.
94. **B**. Equality act.
95. **A**. It is taking action to help people say what they want, secure their rights, represent their interest and obtain the services they need.
96. **A**. Developing the most effective team.
97. **B**. Give assignments clearly taking staff expertise into consideration.
98. **A**. "If you make a mistake with your staff, admit it, apologies and correct the error if possible"
99. **D**. Values, benefits, and work experience that influence their ability to collaborate.
100. **C**. Support groups and alternative medicines.
101. **A**. Mentor.
102. **C**. That she is competent and have required skills.
103. **D**. "It is my responsibility to provide a detailed description of the surgery and ask the patient to sign the consent form".
104. **B**. NMC.
105. **B**. Confidentiality.
106. **C**. Henry Fayol.

# Medicines Management.

107. **D**. Tell him to take one tablet in the morning and one tablet in the evening as ordered.

108. **B.** Pain on movement which is short-lived, with a prescription, when necessary.
**C**. Pain that is intense, unexpected in a location that differs from the previously assessed, needing a review before a prescription is written.
**D**. A patient who has adequately controlled pain relieve with short-lived exacerbation of pain, with a prescription that has 4-hourly frequency of analgesia if necessary.

109. **C**. Hold the medication, document and report.

110. **B**. Slow and shallow breathing, dizziness, sleepiness.

111. **A**. 30 tablets.

112. **B**. Ask patient to hold the breath and bear down.

113. **B.** Advice the colleague to help her.

114. **A**. 150m/hr.

115. **B**. 3 tablets

116. **A**. 2 tablets.

117. **C.** After obtaining blood samples for culture.

118. **A.** Hypnotics.

119. **B**. Sit up and head tilt backwards.

120. **A**. Drink plenty of fluid.

121. **D**. The nurse will have to collaborate with the pharmacist to determine if the capsule is suitable for vegetarians.

122. **A**. Convert administration of drugs to clients is ethically and professionally wrong.

123. **D**. All of the above.

124. **A**. 3 tablets.

125. **C**. 0.5ml.

126. **C**. 0.2ml.

127. **B**. Suspected side effects to blood factor, except immunoglobulin products, **C**. Counterfeit or fake medicines or medical devices.

128. **A**. Blue bag.

129. **A**. Removing from its darkened container exposes the medicine to light and its potency will decrease after 8 weeks.

130. **D**. Dorsogluteal.
131. **B**. Step 2: Opioids for mild to moderate pain.
132. **D**. Anticoagulants
133. **C**. Heart Rate.
134. **D**. Administration of the wrong drug, in the wrong amount, to the wrong patient and or through the wrong route.
135. **D**. None of the above.
136. **A**. As soon as possible after an event has happened to provide current up to date information about the care and condition of the patient or client.
137. **A**. Malignant pleural effusion, **B**. Pneumothorax, **C**. Post-operative conditions such as thoracotomy, cardiac surgery.
138. **E**. All of the above.
139. **A**. Draw a line through error, initial, date and document correct information.
140. **C**. Check the stock of oral morphine sulphate in the CD cupboard with another registered nurse and record this in the control drug book together, check the correct prescription and identity of the patient.
141. **B**. Upper outermost quadrant.
142. **C**. Abbreviations, jargon, meaningless phrases and irrelevant subjective statements.
143. **D**. Yawning, irritability, diaphoresis, cramps and diarrhea
144. **D**. Insomnia.

# Moving and Positioning.

145. **C**. Compartment syndrome.
146. **B**. Sitting up leaning on pillows and inhaling humidified oxygen.
147. **D**. The skeleton provide a structural frame work. This is moved by the muscles that contract or extend and in order to function well it has to cross at least one joint which are attached to the articulating bones.
148. **B**. Offer the patient pain reliever and either use bed scales or a hoist with built in scales.
149. **C**. Push walker forward when using it.
150. **A**. Loss of muscle mass.
151. **B**. Speech therapist.
152. **B**. Slide the walker 10 inches forward then take small steps to maintain balance.
153. **A**. Take long strides.
154. **C**. Crutches and the left leg then advance the right leg.
155. **A**. Make a written report.
156. **A**. Any motion of the limbs or other body parts that pulls away from midline of the body.
157. **A**. Lie the patient supine in bed with the head raised 45-50cm with a backrest.
158. **B**. Hands.
159. **B**. 2 hourly.
160. **C**. 1 each side, 1 at head, then 1 at feet.
161. **B**. If they have a spinal fracture.
162. **B**. Try to diminish increased tenderness by avoiding extra stimulation, ensuring his foot does not come into contact at the edge of the bed; support him with a pillow on his left leg, placed in a lateral position as well as keeping the knee flexed.
163. **D**. To ensure the Spine and Limbs alignment.
164. **D**. Using a four point gait.

## Nutrition, Fluid Balance and Blood Transfusion.

165. **D**. 800 - 2000mls.
166. **C**. Encourage a varied diet as people can react differently.
167. **C**. Group A or O.
168. **C**. 4 to 6 Cups.
169. **D**. Lack of Vitamins.
170. **B**. Intestinal obstruction.
171. **C**. Straining while passing stools.
172. **C**. Accept the client's wish.
173. **C**. High risk of malnutrition.
174. **B**. Diaphoresis, **C**. Cold clammy skin, **D**. Confusion.
175. **A**. Tomatoes, carrots and broccoli.
176. **B**. Testing for the PH of aspirate which should be less than 5.5.
177. **B**. Secondary post-partum hemorrhage.
178. **A**. Severe blood transfusion reaction.
179. **A**. 5%
180. **A**. 83.
181. **A**. Red or maroon-coloured stool rectally.
182. **A**. Self-induced vomiting and she likely has bulimia nervosa.
183. **A**. Blood glucose levels, full blood count, stoma site and bodyweight.
184. **C**. Hypomagnesaemia, **D**. Hypokalemia.
185. **A**. Passing small amount of urine frequently.
186. **D**. The fluid input has exceeded the output.
187. **B**. Sitting upright at 45 to $60^0$
188. **D**. Assessment, source isolation, universal precautions.
189. **C**. Decreased pulse rate.
190. **A**. Dietician.
191. **B**. Abdominal aorta.
192. **A**. The feed.
193. **C**. 1687 (Positive Balance).
194. **B**. Place a sterile bandage or clean cloth and add pressure.

195. **D.** Decreased skin turgor.
196. **A.** Papaya.
197. **D.** Serious adverse reaction.

## Observation
198. **B.** This is a medical emergency. Basic airway, breathing, the circulation should be attended to urgently and help should be sought.
199. **A.** Respiratory rate, bowel movement record and pain assessment and score.
200. **C.** Implied.
201. **A.** Intelligent kindness.
202. **B.** Dermis.
203. Dignity, Empathy, Respect.
204. Economic, Social, Spiritual and Physical care.
205. **B.** Client has brain stem herniation.
206. **A.** Thirst.
207. **A.** Taking care of the airway.
208. **C.** Anaphylactic reaction.
209. **A.** Call the doctor.
210. **A.** Reduced skin turgor.
211. **A.** Has bacterial meningitis. , **B.** Papilledema.
    **C.** Intracranial mass is suspected, **D.** Site skin infection.
212. **A.** Call the doctor.
213. **A.** Every hour.
214. **D.** Bleeding.
215. **A.** Numbness and tingling. **C.** Pain. **D.** Toes swelling
216. **D.** Ketoacidosis.
217. **D.** Diarrhea.
218. **A.** 20.
219. **B.** It is intelligent kindness and is majorly on how people perceive their care.
220. **D.** Urinary Obstruction.
221. **D.** Depression and anxiety, social isolation, loss of independence, exacerbation of symptoms, rapid loss of strength in leg muscles, deconditioning of cardiovascular system leading to increased risk of chest infection, and pulmonary embolism.
222. **C.** 5.

223.    **D**. Sneezing.
224.    **A**. Identifies patient at risk of deterioration.
225.    **D**. Client feel nauseated.

# Patient Comfort and End of Life Care.

226.    **D**. Because of the baroreflex mechanisms which control heart rate and vascular conditions declines with age.

227.    **D**. Cognitive ability, lifestyle, dexterity impairment, position of stoma, skin barrier, type of stoma, consistency of effluent, patient preference.

228.    **C**. Resuscitation.

229.    **C**. Hypertension, smoker, obese men, sedentary lifestyle.

230.    **A**. Tachycardia, vasoconstriction and confusion.

231.    **A**. Care, Compassion, Competence, Communication, Courage, Commitment

232.    **A**. Increasing blood flow velocity in the legs by compression of the deep venous system.

233.    **A**. Dehydration, **B**. Anemia, **C**. Pharma therapeutic agents, **D**. Positional changes in blood pressure and heart rate.

234.    **B**. It will eventually resolve without any medical supervision.

235.    **A**. Tell her to score her pain level, describe its intensity, duration, the site and any relieving measures and what makes it worse, looking for nonverbal clues so that you can determine the appropriate method of pain management.

236.    **B**. Allow the client to go home if he would not pose any threat to himself or others.

237.    **A**. Individualized approach to care.

238.    **D**. Peripheral oedema.

239.    **B**. Alert, voice, pain and unresponsive.

240.    **A**. It is the Initial health care given by a health care provider in a community.

241.    **D**. Abdominal.

242.    **C**. Due to immature T cells.

243.    **A**. Hearing.

244.     **D**. To promote venous flow.
245.     **A**. Directives by the patient himself before dying.
246.     **D**. Yes I will keep the secret because it is confidential.


## Patient Safety.

247.     **A**. Document clearly the reason for not cutting his toe nails and refer him to a chiropodist.
248.     **A**. Contact the pain management team, anesthetist to discuss the situation on how to relieve this condition.
249.     **D**. Help the patient to a safe comfortable position, observe for any injury and report the incident to the nurse in charge, call a doctor. Complete an incident form. At an appropriate time, discuss the incident with the patient and, if they wish, their relatives.
250.     **A**. It is by the law/ order.
251.     **A**. Assess the environment and remove any danger, **B**. Assess for the level of consciousness, **C**. Call for help.
252.     **B**. Place in low fowler's position of 45° angle.
253.     **A**. Cross the wrong entry with a line. Indicating cancellation. Write the date, time, name and signature, document the care given correctly.
254.     **D**. Surgical site infection.
255.     **C**. The care that is focused on the patient.
256.     **A**. Male, female, obese, diabetic, hypertensive, sedentary lifestyle, **C**. Smoker, diabetic and alcoholic, **D**. Male, drug abuse, hypertensive.
257.     **A**. Let the patient go, if he is competent and in his full sense. **C**. If he does not have the mental capacity, restrain the patient and treat.
258.     **A**. Report your concerns immediately, in writing to the appropriate person or body escalating concerns to the NMC, **C**. Ask for advice from your professional body if unsure on what actions to take.


## Pre-operative Care.

259.     **B.** Children under the age of 16 who are believed to have enough intelligence, competence and understanding to fully appreciate what is involved in their treatment and give consent without the need for parental permission.

260.     **A.** Get the patients understanding of the procedure by letting them know the benefits, probably complications stated by the physicians and then they signed the consent that they were well informed.

261.     **C.** Tell the physician that the consent form is not signed.

262.     **D.** To document the details of the procedure in the anaesthetic record.

263.     **A.** Prevent the wound from bleeding.

264.     **C.** Feeding through a radiological inserted gastrostomy(RIG).

265.     **A.** The surgeon.

266.     **D.** To reduce the risk of aspirations, reflux and inhalation of gastric contents.

267.     **C.** This is a normal response to lithium therapy; the patient should be monitored for suicidal behavior.

268.     **B.** He is depressed and he has gone to his earlier state of dependency. He wants the same attention he had received when he was ill.

269.     **C.** Increased energy.

270.     **A.** He has finalized his plan for suicide.

271.     **C.** Regression.

272.     **D.** Make an accurate record of what the person has said to you.

273.     **C.** Denial is a coping mechanism used by an individual with the intention of protecting themselves from painful or distressing information whereas collusion is withholding information from the patient with the intention of protecting them.

274.     **B.** Anxiety has three aspects: Physically, bodily sensations related to flight & fight response, behavioural, such as avoiding the situation, & cognitive (thinking), such as imagining the worst to happen.

275.     **B.** She is repressing anger related to her husband's death.

276.    **D**. Can you tell me about it? "What do you hear about this voices"?

277.    **D**. Repression.

## Respiratory Care.

278.    **D**. Gender.

279.    **A**. A wound dressing change for short- term pain relief or the removal of a chest drain for reduction of anxiety.

280.    **C**. Assess his risk of developing a pressure ulcer with a risk assessment tool. If indicated, admit to an appropriate pressure-relieving mattress and cushion as his bed and chair respectively. Reassess the patient's pressure areas at least twice a day and keep them clean and dry. Review his fluid and nutritional intake and support him to make changes as indicated.

281.    **B**. Arterial blood gas shows the level of Oxygen in the blood and this is part of the patient's care.

282.    **B**. Educating to control the breath by chest Physiotherapist.

283.    **D**. Tongue falling back.

284.    **D**. Increase the level of Oxygen.

285.    **A**. Advise the patient to take measures to quit smoking.

286.    **B**. Retching and vomiting.

287.    **A**. $CO_2$ high, $PO_2$ low.

288.    **D**. Explain to him about advanced directives.

289.    **A**. A prescription requiring, the route, method and duration.

290.    **A**. 70- 110 beats per minute.

291.    **A**. Pneumothorax.

292.    **C**. Airway patency.

293.    **A**. A rare, rapid and disorganized rhythm of heartbeats that rapidly leads to loss of consciousness and sudden death if not treated immediately.

294.    **E**. All of the above.

295.    **B**. 4 – 6.Litres

296.    **D**. All of the above.

297.    **B**. 21%.

298.     **B.** The patient will have a low blood pressure (hypotensive) and will have a fast heart rate (tachycardia) usually associated with skin and mucosal changes.

299.     **B.** Counting the number of respiratory cycles in 1 minutes. One cycle is equal to the complete rise and fall of the patient's chest.

300.     **A.** An initial shock with a manual defibrillator or when prompted by an Automated External Defibrillator (AED).

301.     **B.** Mask.

302.     **A.** Breathing.

303.     **D.** Assess and carry out a full set of observations: blood pressure, respiration rate, oxygen saturation and temperature rhythm, perform a 12 lead ECG. Call the attention of his Physician.

## Vulnerable Adults and Children.

304.     **B.** It includes a range of short-term treatment or rehabilitative services designed to promote independences.

305.     **C.** Remain with the doctor and try to gain confidence of the child and politely assess the child's level of understanding and help the doctor with the information he is looking for.

306.     **C.** A red tray.

307.     **A.** Intervene immediately by halting the staff, make sure that the patient is safe and report to the authority.

308.     **B.** Encourage the patient to stay and rather let his reasons for going out be known.

309.     **C.** Raise a concern and complete a safeguarding form and intervene.

310.     **D.** All of the above.

311.     **C.** Poor nutrition and or fluid intake.

## Wound Management.

312.     **B.** Restorative phase.

313.     **A.** Hot and tender skin.

314.     **A.** 10-24 days.

315.     **A.** Say "I observe you don't seem as usual. Are you sure you are okay?"
316.     **D.** Any type of wound.
317.     **A.** High humidity, non-permeable, conformable, absorbent.
318.     **B.** Open wound showing tissue.
319.     **A.** In the inflammation phase of healing.
320.     **C.** 1 to 5 days.
321.     **D.** Chemical debridement.
322.     **D.** Purulent.
323.     **A.** Transparent film.
324.     **B.** Hemostasis, Inflammation, Proliferation, maturation.
325.     **D.** Holding in place the hydrocolloid dressing for one minute to allow it to adhere.
326.     **C.** Laceration.
327.     **D.** On every wound.
328.     **D.** Adhesive skin closure strips.
329.     **B.** Contaminated wounds.
330.     **A.** Low humidity.

# REFERENCES

Dougherty, L., & Lister S. (2011). The Royal Marsden Manual of Clinical Nursing Proceedure. The Royal Marsden NHS Foundation Trust. (Ed 8; Professional edition). Willey Blackwell.

Dougherty, L., & Lister S. (2015). The Royal Marsden Manual of Clinical Nursing Proceedure. The Royal Marsden NHS Foundation Trust. (Ed 9; Professional edition). Willey Blackwell.

NHS Choices. (2017). Diarrhoea. (Website); www.nhs.uk

National Institute for Health and Care Excellence. (2017). Managing Medicines for adults Receiving Social Care in the Community. (Website); www.nice.org.uk/guidance

Healthy and Safety Executive. (2016). Patient Safety. (Website); www.hse.gov.uk

Nursing and Midwifery Council. (2016).The code for Nurses and Midwives. (Website); www.nmc.org.uk/standards

Nursing and Midwifery Council. (2017). Confidentiality; Disclosure; Raising concern. (Website); www.nmc.org.uk/raisingconcerns

NHS Choices. Consent to treatment. (Website); www.nhs.uk/conditions/consent-to-treatment/pages/children under 16. aspx

NHS Choices. Hypoglycaemia. (Website); https://www.nhs.uk/conditions/hypoglycaemia/pages/Treatment.aspx

https://www.diabetesselfmanagement.com/diabetesresources/definition/metformin/

https://www.nmc.org.uk/about-us/our-role/

https://www.nhsprofessionals.nhs.uk/Download/commsCGS%20.%20Administration%20of%20Medicine%20Guidelines%20V4%20March%202013.pdf

http://www.rpharms.com/support.pdfslpharmaceuticalissuesdosageformsjune.2011.pdf
http://content.digital.nhs.uk/primary.care
user.rcn.com/jkimball.ma.ultranet/...B-and-Tcells.html
www.nhs.uk/cha/pages/2557.aspx?categoryid=72
https://www.nmc.org.uk/standards/code/
www.onh.nhs.uk/sercices/referrals/laboratories/.../specimen-safe-handling.ppt.
www.nursingprocess.org(2016)

www.ingramcontent.com/pod-product-compliance
Lightning Source LLC
Chambersburg PA
CBHW081601220526

45468CB00010B/2730